Handbook of
Essential Antibiotics

GEOFFREY M. SCOTT
*University College Hospital
London, UK*

and

MAY S. KYI
*West Middlesex University Hospital
London, UK*

harwood academic publishers
Australia • Canada • France • Germany • India • Japan
Luxembourg • Malaysia • The Netherlands • Russia • Singapore
Switzerland

Copyright © 2001 OPA (Overseas Publishers Association) N.V. Published by license under the Harwood Academic Publishers imprint, part of The Gordon and Breach Publishing Group.

Amsteldijk 166
1st Floor
1079 LH Amsterdam
The Netherlands

British Library Cataloguing in Publication Data

A catalogue record for this book is available from the British Library.

ISBN 90-5823-176-3 (softcover)

Whilst the information given in this book is believed to be true and accurate at the time of going to press, neither the author nor the publisher can accept any legal responsibility for any injury and/or damage to persons or property as a matter of products liability, negligence or otherwise or from any use or operation of any methods, products, instructions or ideas contained in the material herein. Because of rapid advances in the medical sciences, the publisher recommends that independent verification of diagnoses and drug doses should be made.

CONTENTS

1

INTRODUCTION

There is a bewildering array of antibiotics available in the formulary for treating patients with infections. For some clinical syndromes, such as acute bacterial meningitis, there are very clear indications as to which antibiotic should be used. This is because meningitis is mainly caused by a very small range of organisms whose sensitivities to antibiotics are quite predictable. The choice is determined first, by the need for activity of the antibiotic against the putative or proven organism, secondly by the ability of the antibiotic to penetrate into the brain and cerebrospinal fluid and thirdly by previous clinical experience. Furthermore, the clinical syndrome or preliminary investigations may quite clearly indicate which specific organism is involved. In the case of meningococcal infection, doctors can choose penicillin with a high degree of confidence because there is no resistance. The choice becomes challenging when the patient is reputed to be allergic to penicillin. When there is a chance of resistance as in the case of *Streptococcus pneumoniae*, the choice becomes further complicated. There is always a background anxiety that the meningococcus, like the gonococcus, will eventually develop resistance to penicillins. Penicillin-tolerant or even resistant (a relative term) meningococci have now been described in certain parts of the world but the phenomenon is, at present, so rare as not to influence the choice of penicillin for meningococcal meningitis. The situation is different for gonorrhoea, caused by a closely related organism, where penicillin resistance is so common in the Far East and sub-Saharan Africa, that alternative choices must be made for empirical therapy of urethritis in patients from these parts of the world.

In the UK, antibiotics are not available freely to patients but are available only on prescription by a doctor. In many countries, however, antibiotics are freely available from pharmacies or even from non-professional outlets such as markets. It may be taken for granted that drugs made by *bona fide* pharmaceutical companies are of the correct potency but that is far from the case in the developing world.

A doctor, on evaluating a patient, may come to the conclusion that he has an infection and needs antibiotic treatment. At this stage he relies on history

1

and examination and perhaps immediate tests (e.g. surrogates like the peripheral white cell counts or C-reactive protein) to guide him. He must then 'guess' the diagnosis, 'guess' the likely organism(s) involved and then choose an antibiotic appropriate to this range of organisms. In practice, most doctors tend not to bother with the intermediate steps of wondering which organism might be responsible and simply choose a broad-spectrum antibiotic from a short list on the basis of experience. This is empirical syndromic treatment. If appropriate specimens are sent to the laboratory, after a day or two, an organism might grow and be identified and the decision then is to choose an antibiotic to which the presumptive isolate is likely to be sensitive. The nature of the isolate and its sensitivity are usually known the following day and then specific guided therapy can be recommended by the microbiologist to the clinician. Unfortunately this is rather too late for the patient with a life-threatening infection. In this case, the presumption is that the *sooner* that appropriate antibiotics are given, then the greater likelihood that the infection will be controlled. There seems to be a point of no return in those with serious infections, beyond which no matter how much excellent bactericidal treatment is given, the patient will inevitably succumb because of capillary leakage and organ failure mediated by excessive acute phase response. This then identifies the doctor's dilemma in the use of antibiotics. There is a natural desire to treat patients. Infections are common and giving antibiotics is at least something that physicians can actually *DO*. So there is a low threshold for giving antibiotics and this extends not only to those who are not really very ill but also encourages the use of antibiotics in those who should not be given them at all.

If antibiotics were totally without side effects and there were no ecological disadvantages in the extensive use of antibiotics in man, farm animals and the environment, then the argument that all patients with a cold deserve an antibiotic because they might be brewing bacterial sinusitis, meningitis or pneumonia, would be tenable. But the result of this philosophy is that there is one prescription of antibiotics for each person in the UK for the common cold every year — and virtually all of these are caused by uncomplicated virus infections.

Furthermore, many doctors prescribe antibiotics (e.g. oral cephalosporins or erythromycin) which could have no effect on the evolution of meningitis. Rarely, an experienced doctor will withhold antibiotics because he thinks a patient has a virus infection, but the patient then later dies of meningitis. This is an unanswerable paradox. However, the number of times that antibiotics are given unnecessarily or incorrectly enormously outweighs the number of times that serious infections follow their being withheld. Some have argued that the general usage of antibiotics has resulted in a reduction in a number of diseases such as streptococcal pharyngitis, scarlet fever and post-streptococcal syndromes but there is no evidence for this in the developing world.

Antibiotics all have side-effects, either direct pharmacological ones or allergy or secondary effects on the normal flora, which may be profound. The most devastating of these effects on normal colonising flora in an individual is pseudomembranous colitis which, in its severe form, may be fatal unless colectomy is performed. Minor degrees of gastrointestinal upset occur in perhaps one third of all patients given any antibiotic, a high price to pay for the treatment of a trivial condition. Allergy is usually an inconvenience but may also be fatal.

The effect of antibiotics in selecting resistance in microorganisms over the 50 years that they have been available has been one of the most extraordinary experiments in genetic manipulation.

Within five years of the introduction of penicillin a significant proportion of the *Staphylococcus aureus* isolates were resistant by the production of a penicillinase (β-lactamase). Within a few months of introducing isoniazid and streptomycin, use of either as a single agent for the treatment of tuberculosis led to the emergence of resistant strains. The development of resistance to each new antibiotic introduced is inexorable and inevitable. Vast numbers of microorganisms of many different species live in the upper layers of soil and in the gut of animals. Competition between them leads to an uneasy homeostasis easily upset by climatic changes (in the case of the soil) or introduction of antibiotics or a new pathogen (in the case of gut flora). The predominance of one organism over another is dependent on the natural production of inhibitory substances — a good example being penicillin produced by *Penicillium* moulds which inhibits the growth of many species of naturally occurring bacteria. Microorganisms replicate rapidly and mutations which confer some advantage (e.g. a resistance factor to antibiotics) can be selected with apparent ease. The greatest drive to the selection of such an advantage is the presence of an inhibitory factor. Therefore it is inevitable that the use of antibiotics selects organisms which have adapted to survive.

The influence of antibiotics may be seen in the individual high-dependency patient in whom the exhibition of one agent leads to the emergence of a troublesome resistant organism which may cause infection. Changing practices in medicine have lead to the potential co-existence of, say, *Staphylococcus aureus* and *Staphylococcus epidermidis* associated with implants, enabling transfer of resistance factors from the latter to the former. This is the origin of methicillin-resistant *S. aureus* which is stably resistant and does not appear to be at any particular disadvantage from having the resistance plasmids on board. The presence of antibiotics is not particularly necessary for maintaining colonisation with, for example, methicillin-resistant *S. aureus*, vancomycin-resistant enterococci and multiple-resistant *Salmonella typhimurium*. These organisms may then move from person to person, particularly in the hospital environment but also in the community.

Inevitably, resistant organisms will be seen most often in environments where antibiotics are used prophylactically in the long term and the organisms are not eradicated. Immunosuppressed patients given long term acyclovir develop resistant herpes simplex or given fluconazole, resistant *Candida albicans* or given broad-spectrum antibiotics, resistant pseudomonads.

It is for this reason that some say that, after 50 years, the antibiotic era is nearing an end. There have been no new successful antibiotics directed against a novel target site since pseudomonic acid (mupirocin 1988), which has limited applicability as a topical agent to which resistance has already emerged in methicillin-resistant *Staphylococcus aureus*. Streptogramins and related molecules show promise against resistant Gram positive organisms. Modification of glycopeptides may overcome resistance seen in vancomycin-resistant enterococci. The search for new antibiotics continues apace by examining thousands of novel molecules in screening tests and by dissecting bacterial metabolism in the search for an appropriate novel target. The cynic might say that nature would, in millions of years of evolution under direct competitive pressure for existence, have selected for all the useful antibiotics, and that man has plundered the opportunity and used all the resources available in a mere 50 years. The optimist would say that there are many excellent new antibiotics just around the corner ripe for pharmaceutical development.

Here is a list of antibiotics which we believe are essential, that is, they will have a role which cannot be fulfilled by any other antibiotic from another class. Some would consider the list over-restrictive and others, too liberal. Antibiotic choice is a matter of personal preference and the reader must refer to local guidelines and expert advice. This is very important to establish early on when moving hospitals because the preference of consultants and microbiologists may be quite different.

2

GROUPS OF ANTIBIOTICS: MECHANISMS OF ACTION AND RESISTANCE

Antibiotics can be classified according to their chemical structures, sites of action, their spectrum of activity and whether they are predominantly bactericidal or bacteriostatic. Bactericidal antibiotics kill bacteria, whereas bacteriostatic agents only inhibit their growth and replication. Therefore bacteriostatic antibiotics must rely on the host immune system for eradication of the infection and are ineffective in immunocompromised patients. In practice, infections may be very difficult to eradicate in immunodeficient patients, such as neutropenic patients infected with *Pseudomonas aeruginosa*, even with the most powerful of bactericidal antibiotic combinations.

Many cytotoxic agents kill bacteria but they also kill mammalian cells. Antibiotics must act on pathways unique to bacteria, a phenomenon known as selective toxicity. The following classification is conventional and discusses the drugs according to their sites of action in bacterial metabolism.

CELL WALL ACTIVE GROUPS

β-lactams

Mechanism of action

These bactericidal antibiotics include penicillins, cephalosporins, monobactams and carbapenems. They all interfere with bacterial cell wall biosynthesis eventually leading to lysis and cell death. Unlike mammalian cells, bacteria have a relatively rigid cell wall consisting of a protective framework, peptidoglycan. β-lactam antibiotics are inhibitors of penicillin binding proteins (PBPs), trans- and carboxy-peptidases responsible for catalysing the cross-linking of the peptidoglycan, thus creating a weak cell wall allowing cell lysis. Although all the β-lactam antibiotics have the same mechanism of action, PBPs from different bacteria have different affinities to different penicillins and cephalosporins resulting in varying degrees of susceptibility.

Inhibition of cell wall growth by the action of a β-lactam antibiotic on its own cannot account for the rapid lethality to bacteria. Bacterial cells contain enzymes which synthesise peptidoglycan and autolytic enzymes which are responsible for its breakdown. Autolysin deficient organisms are inhibited but not killed by the β-lactam antibiotics, a phenomenon which is known as tolerance. Persisters are morphologically normal bacteria which survive lethal concentrations of an antibiotic to which it is fully sensitive. β-lactam antibiotics are lethal only to growing cells and a small percentage of the bacteria which are not growing may become persisters as they already have intact cell walls. Once the antibiotic is removed these persisters revert to a normal growth phase. This phenomenon is clearly seen with alpha-haemolytic streptococci in endocarditis.

Many organisms produce β-lactamases which are exported, bind to and inhibit the activity of β-lactam antibiotics. β-lactamase inhibitors are very similar in structure to the β-lactam antibiotics but bind to β-lactamase enzymes with a higher affinity than to the antibiotics themselves, leading to competitive inhibition. Most commercial β-lactamase inhibitors possess only a low level of antibacterial activity, an exception being flucloxacillin often given with penicillin. They are mostly used in combination with more powerful labile antibiotics, preventing their destruction by various β-lactamases produced by the organisms. Plasmid-mediated β-lactamase enzymes (eg. TEM) are readily inhibited by these β-lactamase inhibitors whereas chromosomally-mediated β-lactamases tend to be poorly inhibited.

Penicillins

These consist of acid-stable phenoxymethyl penicillin, orally absorbed, and with a wide spectrum of activity against streptococcal, gonococcal, pneumococcal and meningococcal infections. Benzyl penicillin is the parenteral form, commonly used in hospital practice, to achieve sufficient tissue levels to treat these infections. In addition, it is the drug of choice for a wide variety of infections including actinomycosis, anthrax, diphtheria, gas-gangrene, leptospirosis, syphilis, tetanus, yaws and Lyme disease. Penicillins resistant to staphylococcal β-lactamase include methicillin (not used clinically) and the closely related flucloxacillin and nafcillin. These are used for treating documented penicillin-resistant staphylococcal infections. Sensitive strains of *S. aureus* which do not produce β-lactamase are more sensitive to penicillin than flucloxacillin *in vitro*.

The broader spectrum penicillins such as amoxycillin retain activity against penicillin sensitive organisms but are also active against many Gram negative organisms (such as *Escherichia coli*) and are better absorbed than phenoxymethyl penicillin. They are also inactivated by penicillinases from many bacteria. The spectrum of anti-Gram negative activity is increased in ureidopenicillins (eg azlocillin) but these may be hydrolysed by staphylococcal β-lactamases and enzymes from *Pseudomonas* and *Klebsiella*. Clavulanate inhibits the staphylococcal and some coliform β-lactamases and tazobactam inhibits many β-lactamases from *Pseudomonas* and *Klebsiella*.

Cephalosporins

These are divided into those which are orally active (eg derivatives of cephaloridine) and have some activity against Gram positive organisms such as *Staphylococcus aureus*, those which can only be given parenterally (eg cefuroxime) but are more active against Gram negatives, and those, again mostly only parenterally active, which are active against *Pseudomonas* and resistant *Klebsiella* (eg ceftazidime) and marginally active against Gram positives.

Carbapenems

Imipenem and meropenem have a very broad spectrum of activity so are commonly used to treat serious infections empirically. *Stenotrophomonas maltophilia* is usually resistant, so this tends to be selected as an important colonising organism in units where carbapenems are widely used.

Mechanisms of resistance

Resistance to β-lactam antibiotics is due to:

- a change in the affinity of the penicillin binding proteins or
- failure to reach the target receptor site (usually by changes in the permeability of Gram negative cell membranes or active export by the cells) or
- the production of β-lactamase enzymes which hydrolyse these antimicrobials before they can reach their target. β-lactamases are either produced in great excess in the milieu surrounding an organism, as in the case of staphylococcal penicillinases, or produced in rather lower levels sufficient to inactivate antibiotics within the periplasmic space between the outer membrane and cell wall of Gram negative bacteria.

Any of these resistance mechanisms may be determined by DNA coding for proteins on chromosomes or plasmids. Plasmids are small circular lengths of DNA distinct from the chromosome which are reproduced with bacterial replication and may be transferred between bacteria within species or from one species to another. R(resistance)-factor is the term used for plasmids which carry a family of resistance genes, which can immediately transfer multiple resistance to progeny or even to new strains or species of bacteria. Transposons are DNA elements which appear to enhance transmission of resistance factors and incorporation of plasmid into chromosomal DNA. Resistance may be transmitted directly from one bacterium to another via type II pili or by bacteriophages.

Glycopeptides

Mechanism of action

These bactericidal antibiotics inhibit bacterial cell wall synthesis by binding to the peptide chains disrupting the cross-linking of peptidoglycan. Glycopeptides bind rapidly and irreversibly to the d-Ala-dAla complex of peptidoglycan inhibiting cell wall synthesis. Glycopeptides are active against Gram positive aerobes and anaerobes.

Mechanism of resistance

- The porins of Gram negative bacteria are impermeable to these antibiotics because of their size.
- Alteration of target

Almost all Gram positive organisms are susceptible to glycopeptides with the exception of *Staphylococcus haemolyticus*, which is intrinsically resistant to teicoplanin. While *Leuconostoc*, *Lactobacillus* and *Erysipelothrix* spp. are resistant to vancomycin, some *Enterococcus* spp. are resistant to either or both teicoplanin and vancomycin. This resistance is chromosomally mediated via a complex family of genes (eg Van A and Van B) which code for fundamental changes in the peptide structure of peptidoglycan (eg d-Ala-dAla to a-Ala-d-Lac).

- Vancomycin tolerant *Staphylococcus aureus* (MIC 8 mg/l) has a thick wall and altered penicillin binding proteins.

PROTEIN SYNTHESIS INHIBITORS

Aminoglycosides

Mechanism of action

Aminoglycosidic aminocyclitols (commonly called aminoglycosides) are the only bactericidal drugs among the many agents which inhibit bacterial protein synthesis. They act by binding to the 30S subunit of the ribosome resulting in misreading of the genetic message. They may also inhibit the initiation and elongation reactions of the protein synthesis. Cell death occurs due to the accumulation of abnormal initiation complexes.

These agents are not absorbed so must be given parenterally for systemic infection but they may also be used orally for their effects on gut flora. Topical preparations are also available but may cause sensitisation and resistance. The first to come into clinical use was streptomycin, now reserved for anti-tuberculosis regimens because it is rather toxic and does not have very good activity against many other bacteria. Gentamicin is the cheapest and most popular aminoglycoside but resistance to this antibiotic is now quite common so amikacin is preferred in many units. Less toxic antibiotics with virtually the same activity as gentamicin are tobramycin and netilmicin but they are substantially more expensive to give and monitor. Spectinomycin is a true aminoglycoside and reserved for the second-line treatment of gonorrhoea. In addition to the usual mechanism of action of the aminoglycosides, spectinomycin also produces alterations in the surface morphology of the gonococcus resulting in cell lysis, probably accounting for its perceived value as a single dose treatment in this infection.

Mechanisms of resistance

Bacterial resistance to aminoglycosides may be due to:

- specific inactivating enzymes (eg. acetylating, adenylating and phosphorylating) which are usually R plasmid mediated, conjugate the aminoglycoside to an acetyl group, an adenylyl group or a phosphoryl group, rendering them inactive.

There is a large family of inactivating enzymes which have more or less specificity against individual members of the group. Amikacin tends to be more resistant to enzymic degradation than others in this group. The prevalence of individual aminoglycoside-inactivating enzymes varies widely and it is difficult to predict the precise enzymologic mechanism responsible for aminoglycoside resistance in an individual isolate.

- genetic mutation resulting in a change in the 30S ribosomal subunit, leading to decreased ribosomal binding of the drug.

Ribosomal resistance is uncommon and is only recognised in streptomycin.

- alteration of the Gram negative bacterial cell membrane permeability.

Aminoglycosides are inactive under anaerobic conditions due to reduction in the transport of these drugs into the bacterial cell.

- alteration of the ribosomal structure of the gonococcus accounts for resistance to spectinomycin.

Chloramphenicol

Mechanism of action

Chloramphenicol inhibits bacterial protein synthesis by binding to the 50S ribosomal subunit and preventing peptide bond formation. This is a bacteriostatic antibiotic, but in high concentrations and in certain conditions such as typhoid fever, chloramphenicol appears to be bactericidal.

Mechanisms of resistance

Chloramphenicol resistance is due to:

- the production of a plasmid mediated enzyme, chloramphenicol acetyl transferase, which inactivates the drug, or
- Alterations in the cell outer membrane permeability may be the cause of constitutive resistance in *Pseudomonas aeruginosa*. Changes in outer membrane porins can be coded for by transposons which are special segments of DNA which can transpose from one plasmid to another or to the bacterial chromosome.

Macrolides/lincosamines

Mechanism of action

Though structurally unrelated to each other, these important antimicrobials bind to the 50S ribosomal subunit, inhibiting the translocation reaction in the macrolides and inhibiting peptide bond formation in the lincosamines. The binding sites overlap with each other and also with that of chloramphenicol. Lincosamines bind only to the 50S ribosomal subunit of Gram positive organisms and Gram negative anaerobes. Gram negative bacilli tend to be resistant to macrolides due to their inability to penetrate the cell membrane. Macrolides tend to be bacteriostatic *in vitro,* but *in vivo* they are bactericidal in higher concentrations.

The macrolides include erythromycin, which is predominantly active against Gram positive pyogenic organisms and some unusual Gram negatives such as *Bordetella pertussis* and *Campylobacter* spp., and the recently introduced clarithromycin (notable for enhanced activity against *Haemophilus* spp.), while azithromycin has a 16-membered ring structure and is termed an azolide. The latter has a broader spectrum even than clarithromycin and useful pharmacokinetics which allow successful treatment with small numbers of doses. Macrolides are particularly useful for treating atypical pneumonia caused by *Mycoplasma pneumoniae, Legionella pneumophila, Coxiella burnetii* and *Chlamydia psittaci.* Of the lincosamines, clindamycin is the most useful being orally bioavailable and is very useful for bone and soft tissue infections and inhalational pneumonitis which usually involves mouth flora.

Mechanism of resistance

Resistance to macrolides may be due to:

- reduced ribosomal affinity to macrolides (plasmid-mediated) or
- the production of inactivating enzymes or
- impermeability of the outer membrane of Gram negative bacteria
- active excretion

'Dissociated resistance' in *Staphylococcus aureus* isolates has been described between erythromycin and clindamycin. This mechanism is due to an alteration in the ribosomal RNA reducing the affinity of binding between macrolides and the ribosomes. Inducible resistance of this kind is found in certain staphylococci and streptococci. In practice, if *S. aureus* is resistant to erythromycin but appears sensitive to clindamycin *in vitro*, it will almost certainly be resistant to clindamycin *in vivo,* but the same may not apply to other organisms.

Tetracyclines

Mechanism of action

After a complex energy dependent mechanism of entry into the cell, these antibiotics bind to the 30S ribosomal subunit and inhibit protein synthesis in the organism. They may also cause alterations in the cytoplasmic membrane leading to leakage of intracellular products.

Earlier tetracyclines (oxytetracycline, etc) have been eclipsed by those with a longer duration of action and fewer side-effects (minocycline and doxycycline). Tetracyclines are useful for acne, atypical pneumonia, for *Haemophilus influenzae* in exacerbations of chronic bronchitis and some unusual infections.

Mechanisms of resistance

Resistance to tetracyclines is due to

- decreased uptake and/or (commonly) increased efflux of the antibiotic leading to decreased concentration within the bacterial cell, or

- the synthesis of novel envelope located proteins, a mechanism only found in the Gram negative bacteria.

Bacterial resistance to tetracyclines can be transferred on plasmids or by transposons.

Fusidic acid

Mechanism of action

This is a steroid which binds to the 50S ribosomal subunit inhibiting bacterial protein synthesis. It acts by stabilising the ribosome-G-GTP complex, thus preventing the recycling of factor G, resulting in the accumulation of undissociated complexes which interfere with bacterial replication.

Mechanism of resistance

Resistance is mainly due to

- mutation causing alteration in factor G
- Gram negative bacteria are resistant due to the impermeability of the outer cell membrane.

Although it has a fairly broad-spectrum of action including many anaerobes, fusidic acid is used almost exclusively for treating staphylococcal infection. It has a property of penetrating pus well and therefore has an advantage over flucloxacillin. However, this antimicrobial should be used in combination with other antibiotics to prevent the emergence of resistance.

DNA SYNTHESIS INHIBITORS

Folate antagonists

The antibacterial folate antagonists constitute the sulphonamides and trimethoprim.

Mechanism of action

Sulphonamides are structurally similar to p-aminobenzoic acid (PABA) and inhibit the enzyme dihydropteroate synthetase which is essential for the earlier part of the bacterial folic acid synthesis. They may also act independently on the dihydrofolate reductase (DHFR), the enzyme essential for the final stage of the folic acid synthesis. Trimethoprim is an inhibitor of dihydrofolate reductase only. Neither antibiotic significantly inhibits the mammalian folic acid synthesis enzymes except in very high concentrations.

Sulphamethoxazole in combination with trimethoprim, known as co-trimoxazole, is possibly bactericidal and may have synergistic activity against micro-organisms although this is controversial. However, sulphonamides and trimethoprim are bacteriostatic. Trimethoprim alone is the most commonly selected first choice for urinary infection. Considerable concern has been shown about the severe hypersensitivity reactions to sulphonamides so they should be reserved for the treatment of a few specific infections such as *Pneumocystis carinii* and nocardiasis. Many sulphonamides were made including long-acting and non-absorbable variants but they are mostly not available now. Sulphonamides penetrate the blood-brain barrier well so are useful in meningitis but there is so much resistance in the common organisms that other antibiotics are generally favoured initially. Co-trimoxazole is useful for *Pneumocystis carinii* infections in AIDS.

Mechanisms of resistance

Some bacterial species are intrinsically resistant to trimethoprim because of poor penetration or because they contain DHFR with a reduced affinity for trimethoprim.

Acquired resistance to sulphonamides may be:

● chromosomal, leading either to a less susceptible dihydropteroate synthetase or over-production of para-aminobenzoate.
● R plasmid mediated resulting in altered dihydropteroate synthetase.

Acquired resistance to trimethoprim may be due to:

● chromosomal mutation leading either to impaired penetration of the organism by trimethoprim, or the production of the dihydrofolate reductase with reduced sensitivity to trimethoprim.
● R plasmid mediated resistance which confers high level resistance either due to production of trimethoprim-resistant dihydrofolate reductase, or production of enzyme with a reduced affinity for trimethoprim.

Quinolones

Mechanism of action

This group of bactericidal antimicrobials inhibit the A subunit of DNA gyrase, an enzyme necessary for supercoiling bacterial DNA, allowing it to fit into the cell. The newer fluoro-quinolones penetrate the outer membrane of Gram negative organisms better than nalidixic acid.

Nalidixic acid became the favoured quinolone before fluoroquinolones were introduced but is now obsolete. It was used mainly for urinary infections but fluorination enhanced the spectrum of activity to such an extent that the new derivatives were more active against Gram negative organisms and uniquely useful as orally-active anti-pseudomonal agents, active in single dose against penicillin-resistant gonorrhoea and with excellent efficacy in typhoid fever. There are many fluoroquinolones some with enhanced activity against Gram positive bacteria, some with better bioavailibility. They all have modest anti-mycobacterial activity so are useful as part of combination chemotherapy against *Mycobacterium avium intracellulare*.

Mechanisms of resistance

Three mechanisms are associated with quinolone resistance:

- a change in the genes coding for DNA gyrase or topoisomerase IV or
- a change in the outer membrane porins.

These two mechanisms are due to chromosomal mutation. With the earlier quinolones (eg nalidixic acid), the development of resistance while on treatment was a problem. This effect is not so common with the newer fluoro-quinolones but it may be seen while treating organisms such as *Pseudomonas aeruginosa* in protected sites. No transferable resistance has been convincingly demonstrated.

- active efflux of the agent from the bacterial cell.

Nitroimidazoles

Mechanism of action

The mechanism of action of this group of antimicrobials is thought to be on the bacterial DNA causing extensive strand breakage under reducing conditions. The reduction products of the imidazoles, produced by the action of anaerobic bacterial nitroreductases, are also thought to be responsible for the killing effects.

Metronidazole has activity against many organisms with entirely or part anaerobic metabolism. The spectrum is wide, encompassing most anaerobic bacteria and some protozoa, notably *Entamoeba histolytica*.

Mechanism of resistance

Aerobic organisms are not inhibited by metronidazole.

Anaerobic organisms resistant to nitroimidazoles are uncommon but resistance may be due to

- lower activity of nitroreductases in anaerobic bacteria (eg *Bacteroides fragilis*).

Rifamycins

Mechanism of action

This family of closely related antibiotics inhibits the synthesis of DNA-dependent RNA polymerase in bacteria. They are very active against most Gram positive bacteria, particularly staphylococci, bactericidal to mycobacteria and active against some Gram negatives including *Neisseria* spp. (meningococcus and gonococcus), *Brucella* and *Legionella* spp.. Rifamycin derivatives are also active against some DNA viruses *in vitro* but have never been developed for this application.

Rifampicin is commonly used for treating tuberculosis and leprosy. Rifabutin (a derivative of rifamycin S) and rifapentin have better pharmacokinetics, in particular a longer duration of action, and may kill atypical mycobacteria (eg *M. avium*) rather better. Rifampicin may be used to treat resistant staphylococcal infections. Selection of resistant mutants of *S. aureus* or *M. tuberculosis* occurs rapidly.

Mechanism of resistance

This is due to

- the mutation of the β subunit of the DNA-dependent RNA polymerase resulting in altered binding site for the drug.

Rapid emergence of chromosomally determined resistant mutants occur with rifamycins so they should not be used alone.

Nitrofurans

Mechanism of action

The exact mechanism of action is not known but they cause both single and double DNA strand breakage. They also have a direct effect on protein synthesis. Nitrofurantoin is considerably less active at alkaline pH (as induced in the urine by *Proteus* spp. or in renal tubular acidosis).

Nitrofurantoin is concentrated in the urine and is not active against infections elsewhere. It is active against most urinary pathogens.

Mechanism of resistance

- Resistance is due to a reduction in nitrofuran reductase activity. Resistance may be chromosomally or R plasmid determined.

ANTI-MYCOBACTERIAL AGENTS

Most conventional antibiotics have no activity against mycobacteria which have a special cell wall making them resistant to penetration. However, the mycolic acids are a target for some uniquely active drugs like isoniazid. Broad spectrum drugs active against mycobacteria include rifamycins, streptomycin, macrolides and quinolones. SEE rifampicin.

Isoniazid

Mechanism of action

Isoniazid (isonicotinic acid/hydrazide) is bactericidal to *Mycobacterium tuberculosis*, blocking mycolate synthetase, an enzyme which is unique to mycobacteria, so inhibiting the synthesis of mycolic acids which are part of the outer cell wall structure.

This antibiotic is key to the treatment of tuberculosis, but resistance is fairly common worldwide and is constitutive in most strains of *M. avium* causing clinical disease in AIDS patients, as well as in other atypical species.

Mechanism of resistance

- Occurs under selective antimicrobic pressure of constitutively less susceptible variants of *M. tuberculosis*.
- Some strains resist uptake of the drug.
- Other molecular basis

Most resistant strains are naturally occuring mutants, the evolution of which is potentiated by the use of a single agent in the treatment of mycobacterial disease. This is known as secondary or acquired drug resistance.

Primary drug resistance may be present in patients not previously exposed to isonazid and is common in the developing countries of South-East Asia (15%), Africa and certain parts of USA. Atypical mycobacteria are usually resistant to isoniazid.

Pyrazinamide

Mechanism of action

This is an effective bactericidal anti-tuberculosis drug, with a specific sterilising action against *M. tuberculosis* in the intracellular environment of the macrophages, but the precise mechanism of action is unknown.

Mechanism of resistance

- *M. bovis* is intrinsically resistant to the drug and atypical mycobacteria are also usually resistant but the exact mechanism of resistance is not known.

Ethambutol

Another unique bacteriostatic anti-tuberculosis agent of uncertain action probably acting on RNA synthesis.

This is often used as part of a combination not necessarily to enhance anti-mycobacterial activity but mainly to prevent the emergence of resistance to, say, rifampicin when an organism is already resistant to isoniazid at the start of treatment.

Mechanism of resistance

Although primary resistance has been reported, the exact mechanism is not known. Resistance is selected if the drug is used alone but ethambutol is very effective at preventing the emergence of resistance to rifampicin. The combination of rifampicin and ethambutol is valuable for treating *M. kansasii* infections.

SECOND LINE ANTI-TUBERCULOSIS AGENTS

These include aminoglycosides (particularly streptomycin, kanamycin and amikacin), quinolones, some macrolides, cycloserine, ethionamide and prothionamide, thiacetazone (widely used in Africa as first line agent), a polypeptide antibiotic called capreomycin and para-aminosalicyclic acid (not currently manufactured). All but the aminoglycosides are relatively poor anti-tuberculosis agents compared with the first line drugs (rifampicin, isoniazid and streptomycin), are more toxic and regimens are complicated, untested and unproven.

3

IMPORTANT PROPERTIES OF ANTIBIOTICS

SPECTRUM OF ACTION

The spectrum of activity of an antibiotic is its most important property from the point of view of choosing a drug for empirical therapy. Gram negative organisms differ from Gram positives in having an extra bi-lamellar membrane exterior to the peptidoglycan cell wall. Nutrients and waste products must pass through this membrane through protein organelles called porins. Large molecules (eg glycopeptides) cannot get through porins so Gram negative organisms are all resistant to glycopeptides but passage through the porins may also be restricted by the charge of some small but polar antibiotics. Metabolism may also determine susceptibility to antibiotics, the best example being the unique susceptibility of anaerobes to metronidazole. Some organisms have unique targets for certain antibiotics while others have enzyme systems with low affinity for the antibiotics which appears to confer resistance on these bacteria. For example, aztreonam (a monobactam) is surprisingly only active against Gram negatives.

CLINICAL USEFULNESS

There may be considerable disparity between the *in vitro* activity of a drug and its usefulness and applicability in clinical disease. A drug may be highly active but may simply not penetrate to the site of infection. Mupirocin is inactivated if given systemically but is highly active topically. Nitrofur-antoin is concentrated more in the urine or in the renal tissue depending on the pH of the urine, but it is not distributed in other compartments of the body sufficient to have any effect in systemic infection. An antibiotic may not act in the presence of unfavourable conditions, such as pus (aminoglycosides) or in an alkaline urine (nitrofurantoin). Many antibiotics are highly active against *Salmonella typhi in vitro* but many, the aminoglycosides and cephalosporins being good examples, simply do not work in clinical typhoid. Perhaps this is because of the intracellular site of this organism. Certainly discrepancy between *in vitro* and *in vivo* activity is most often seen with intracellular organisms such as *Legionella pneumophila*. In legionellosis, effective antibiotic regimens (eg erythromycin or erythromycin plus rifampicin) have been discovered by anecdotal clinical experience but have never been evaluated in a proper controlled trial.

PHARMACOKINETICS

This concerns absorption, distribution, metabolism, and excretion but the critical feature of the pharmacology of any antimicrobial agent is its delivery to the site of infection in a concentration which exceeds the minimal inhibitory or cidal concentration of that antibiotic for the organism in question. Drugs like erythromycin, oral cephalosporins, penicillin, aminoglycoside and glycopeptides do not penetrate the CSF so are ineffective in meningitis even though they may be very active against the organism involved *in vitro*. The duration of action is important and an important specific property of antimicrobials in this respect is the tendency for the inhibitory effect of an antimicrobial to persist after the concentration has fallen below the *in vitro* inhibitory concentration. This is known as the post-antibiotic effect, and may indicate successful less frequent dosing intervals.

In the serum an antibiotic may be more or less protein bound and this may influence distribution in the tissues and persistence. Many antibiotics are metabolised, often in the liver and are involved in enterohepatic circulation. Antibiotics and their metabolites which may be inactive or more active than the parent compound are usually excreted through the kidneys but a few are cleared predominantly through the liver. Knowledge of biliary and urinary concentrations will determine choice for infections at these sites. Failure of these organs will influence choice and dosage of the drugs. Some drugs are cleared by renal replacement methods, others (eg glycopeptides) are not cleared at all. A few compounds (eg rifampicin) are concentrated in the respiratory secretions.

CHOICE OF DOSE

For years there have been controversies about the dosage of drugs. Empirical dosage used to be used and dose-ranging studies were rarely done. Intelligent extrapolation from pharmacokinetic results may give a more reasonable clue. However, pharmacokinetics are often altered in ill patients. Furthermore a drug company will want to license a drug at the dose which has been used in all studies (or some, if not all, the trials will have to be repeated). There is little if any encouragement to find the minimum effective dose. Important exceptions are gonorrhoea, a clear clinical syndrome with easily measured endpoints (patient clinically better and no bacteria cultivable after treatment). Yet doing trials in gonorrhoea is fraught with difficulty because of lack of patient compliance.

When antibiotics were first introduced, the dose was chosen by guess work and inadequate doses were suggested by treatment failure. Some drugs can be easily monitored in the serum (aminoglycosides, glycopeptides and some antifungals). Blood levels can predict tissue levels to a certain extent but much of this monitoring is to reduce the risk of toxicity rather than to ensure efficacy. Providing the dose leads to a concentration of antibiotic in tissues which is a low multiple of the minimal inhibitory or cidal concentration of that antibiotic against that bacterium, then giving more cannot kill the bacteria faster or more effectively. Sometimes the dose is increased because there is likely to be a poor concentration gradient from blood into an infected lesion (as in infective endocarditis). Alternatively an organism such as *Pseudomonas aeruginosa* may be relatively resistant. Dosage regimens are now mostly based on some pharmacological indices backed up by, in the main, very inadequate clinical trials. In general though, the widely held perception that MORE ANTIBIOTIC MUST KILL BETTER and therefore that ILL PATIENTS NEED MORE ANTIBIOTIC is not correct.

PHARMACODYNAMICS

Perhaps the most scientific method of deciding on dose and dose frequency is pharmacodynamic modelling which is prerequisite for the development of a new drug. The relevant measures are concentration of the free antibiotic in serum over time after the dose (given by the area under the curve) or the maximal serum concentration (Cmax) as a ratio of the MIC for the organism in question. The post antibiotic effect will also be factored in. Equivalent modelling can be used for concentrations of antibiotics in tissues such as skin blebs in volunteers or surgical specimens, or extrapolation of distribution kinetics of labelled drug in animals.

LENGTH OF A COURSE

It is not possible to predict the course of an infection so the length of treatment should not be didactically stated at the start of therapy. In general practice, a single dose of antibiotic will cure 70% of uncomplicated urinary infections and if it does not, a very long course may be indicated. For respiratory infections it is hardly worth continuing antibiotics for more than 5 days. Recommendations that 'a course of antibiotics must be finished' were made on the theoretical basis that too short a course might select for resistance but this seems unlikely. In neutropenic patients with *Pseudomonas* bacteraemia, antibiotics should be continued until the white cell count begins to recover even though the patient may be afebrile. Meningococcal infection in sub-Saharan Africa is as effectively treated by single doses of intramuscular penicillin as many days of high dose intravenous penicillin used in the UK. On the other hand, *Streptococcus pneumoniae* tends to persist in pus in the meninges relatively inaccessible to antibiotics and may grow again if penicillin is stopped too early. The only clear guidelines on length of treatment course are for urinary tract infections (a single dose of some antibiotics will cure 70% of UTIs) and tuberculosis where a powerful combination regimen will cure about 70% in 4 months but about 98% in six months. In hospital, antibiotic prescriptions should be reviewed daily asking the question 'why should I **not** stop antibiotics today?'.

SIDE EFFECTS

Theoretically, because antibiotics work on enzyme systems unique to micro-organisms, they should rarely cause direct pharmacological effects in mammalian cell systems but in practice this is not so. Common side effects of all antimicrobials include rashes, fever, nausea, vomiting and diarrhoea. They are very common. These unwanted effects are either direct pharmacologic properties or, perhaps more importantly, effects on the normal colonising bacterial flora. Simple effects of broad spectrum antibiotics on lactobacilli in the vagina and on mouth flora can lead to the overgrowth of *Candida* spp. An effect on the normal large bowel flora can allow the proliferation of *Clostridium difficile*, and if a toxin producer, resultant diarrhoea or pseudomembranous colitis. Within a short time of taking oral broad spectrum antibiotics, coliforms appear in the mouth and can contribute to mucositis. It may take weeks or even months for the coliforms to disappear and for the normal flora to re-establish.

CONTRAINDICATIONS

Generally, an absolute contraindication is previous type I hypersensitivity (anaphylaxis) to a specific antibiotic. There are some states, particularly pregnancy, where certain drugs are contraindicated because of teratogenic or other important metabolic or pharmacologic effects. Doctors should be wary of drugs which accumulate in the presence of deranged renal (aminoglycosides and glycopeptides) and liver (macrolides) function and which then might contribute to worsening disease.

DRUG INTERACTIONS

Some antimicrobials have important interactions with other drugs which may or may not be antimicrobials. Some antibiotics antagonise each other, the classical example being penicillin and chloramphenical against *Streptococcus pneumoniae*. Others synergise, that is the total activity is considerably greater than the sum of the individual activities. Aminoglycosides synergise with β-lactam antibiotics in the treatment of streptococcal, coliform and *Pseudomonas* infections. Penicillin and aminoglycosides are incompatible in the same intravenous solution. Antibiotics may either facilitate or decrease the excretion of other drugs, thus affecting their activity, an effect on metabolic enzymes or on a common pathway of drug absorption or excretion. The effects of rifampicin on the metabolism of corticosteroids, the contraceptive pill and warfarin are profound. Tetracyclines are chelated by calcium in milk or antacids and are then not absorbed from the gastrointestinal tract.

SELECTION OF RESISTANCE

Some antibiotics, such as fusidic acid or rifampicin, used alone will select resistant mutants. Otherwise, in hospital practice, use of a broad spectrum antibiotic will kill much of the normal flora, such that the patient is susceptible to new hospital-associated bacteria which inevitably will be resistant to the antibiotic used. This is often seen in ill patients on ventilators or with continuing intra-abdominal sepsis.

COST

New antibiotics cost more than old ones because of the inflationary nature of development costs. A new antibiotic will first find itself in the formulary of the hospitals where trials were performed. Unless it has a unique property (such as ciprofloxacin being orally active against *Pseudomonas* spp.) the introduction of a new drug into the formulary will depend on minor advantages and cost will be a major determinant.

4

ESSENTIAL ANTIBIOTICS

Essential antibiotics have a unique role not fulfilled by any other (cheaper or well-established) drug.

DRUGS ESSENTIAL IN THE FORMULARY AND THEIR UNIQUE INDICATION(S)

Amikacin	Gentamicin-resistant Gram-negatives and some resistant mycobacterial infections.
Amoxicillin	Continuation of oral treatment for endocarditis. Oral treatment of sensitive organisms (eg *Streptococcus pyogenes, Streptococcus pneumoniae*, gonorrhoea, urinary infections, etc).
Second-generation	cephalosporin (eg cefuroxime) Broad spectrum for Gram negative infections.
Third-generation	cephalosporin (eg ceftazidime) *Pseudomonas* spp. and resistant Gram-negative infections.
Chloramphenicol	Broad spectrum, meningitis, brain abscess.
Ciprofloxacin	Typhoid, *Pseudomonas* spp. infections and penicillin-resistant gonorrhoea.
Clindamycin	Inhalation pneumonitis and osteomyelitis. *Mycoplasma hominis* in pregnancy and lactation. Anaerobic infections.
Co-trimoxazole	*Pneumocystis carinii* pneumonia.
Doxycycline	Atypical pneumonia and *Chlamydia trachomatis*.
Erythromycin	Atypical pneumonia. *Chlamydia* in pregnancy.
Flucloxacillin	*Staphylococcus aureus*.
Fusidic acid	*Staphylococcus aureus*.
Gentamicin	Serious Gram-negative and -positive infections.
Isoniazid	Tuberculosis.
Metronidazole	Anaerobic infection. Amoebiasis.
Penicillin	Sensitive infections (eg *Streptococcus pyogenes*, meningococcus, pneumococcus).
Pyrazinamide	Tuberculosis.

Rifampicin   Tuberculosis and *Staphylococcus aureus* infections.
Teicoplanin   Resistant Gram-positive infections.
Trimethoprim   Urinary infection, staphylococcal infections (with
                    rifampicin).

OPTIONAL ANTIMICROBIAL DRUGS

Azithromycin   Single dose treatment of *Chlamydia* spp. infections.
First generation cephalosporin (eg cephalexin)   Sensitive urinary infections.
Second-generation cephalosporin (eg cefotaxime, ceftriaxone)   Extended
                    spectrum anti-Gram-negative infection. Meningitis.
Clarithromycin   *Mycobacterium avium* complex and alternative to
                    erythromycin.
Co-amoxiclav   Extension of activity of amoxycillin to include some β-
                    lactamase producing strains.
Ethambutol   Resistant tuberculosis.
Imipenem   Resistant Gram-negative and anaerobic infections.
Mupirocin   Topical activity against staphylococci and streptococci.
Nitrofurantoin   Urinary infection.
Piperacillin and tazobactam   Resistant Gram-negative infections.
Quinupristin–dalfopristin   Resistant Gram-positive infections.
Spectinomycin   Penicillin-resistant gonorrhoea.
Sulphonamide   Nocardiasis.
Tetracycline   Acne, etc.
Vancomycin   Resistant Gram-positive infections (eg *Staphylococcus
                    haemolyticus*).

AMIKACIN

Antibiotic group

Aminoglycoside

Spectrum

Active against many Gram-negative and some Gram-positive aerobic
bacteria; also active against *Mycobacterium tuberculosis* and other atypical
mycobacteria including some strains of *Mycobacterium avium* complex.
Little activity against anaerobes.

Clinical usefulness

Useful in the treatment of serious Gram-negative infections resistant to
gentamicin. It acts synergistically with other antibacterials such as beta-lactams,

cephalosporins and quinolones. It is also used as combination therapy in the treatment of resistant tuberculosis and *Mycobacterium avium* complex infection.

Preparations available

Parenteral only, intravenous preferred.

Usual adult dose

15 mg/kg (iv infusion) daily in 2–3 divided doses
Once daily dosage of amikacin can be given (see gentamicin).

References

Beringer PM, Vinks AA, Jelliffe RW. Pharmacokinetics of once-daily amikacin dosing in patients with cystic fibrosis. *Journal of Antimicrobial Chemotherapy* 1998,**41**:142–144
Van Haeverbeek M, Siska G, Herchuelz A. Pharmacokinetics of once daily amikacin in elderly patients. *Journal of Antimicrobial Chemotherapy* 1993;**31**:185–7

Pharmacology

Not absorbed from the gastrointestinal tract but after parenteral administration, widely distributed mainly in the extracellular fluids and the kidneys. Like all aminoglycosides, it penetrates poorly into the CSF and bronchial secretions. Amikacin is excreted entirely as active unchanged form through the kidneys.

Monitoring

Peak and trough drug levels should be checked either with the third or the fifth dose to assess accumulation to reduce the risk of renal failure and ototoxicity. A trough level (optimally <5 mg/L) should be taken immediately prior to the next dose and peak level (15–25 mg/L) one hour after completion of infusion. A single daily dosage of amikacin has been evaluated as for gentamicin and netilmicin.

Side effects

See gentamicin. Amikacin may be more likely to cause ototoxicity and renal impairment than gentamicin but a direct controlled comparison has not been done.

Contraindications

See gentamicin

Drug interactions

See gentamicin

Other similar drugs

See gentamicin.

Kanamycin (from which amikacin is derived and is used only for tuberculosis), netilmicin, tobramycin. Liposome-encapsulated amikacin is under development with the hope of lowered toxicity for equivalent activity.

Reference

Leitzke S, Bucke W, Borner K, Muller R, Hahn H, Ehlers S. Rationale for and efficacy of prolonged-interval treatment using liposome-encapsulated amikacin in experimental *Mycobacterium avium* infection. *Antimicrobial Agents and Chemotherapy* 1998;**42**:459–461

AMOXICILLIN

Antibiotic group

β-lactam with activity against Gram positive organisms which are sensitive to penicillin and some Gram-negative organisms but not *Klebsiella, Enterobacter, Serratia* or *Pseudomonas* spp.

Spectrum

Wide spectrum against Gram-positive, Gram-negative and anaerobic bacteria.

Usefulness

Only useful for the treatment of certain specific syndromes or micro-biologically proved infections. Exceptions are conditions where there is little or no resistance (eg Group A *Streptococcus* in throat or soft tissues). Amoxicillin is also useful for treating sensitive enterococcal infections and synergises with aminoglycosides for this indication; therefore useful with gentamicin for gall bladder sepsis. Otherwise, usefulness in empirical treatment of urinary infections and gonorrhoea (in some parts of the world) is much eroded by resistance. Amoxicillin 3 g is used with probenecid 1 g as oral eradicative treatment of gonorrhoea when there is a low expectation of resistance but this treatment is not active against *Chlamydia trachomatis*. It is also used in listeriosis often in combination with gentamicin and in the continuation phase in endocarditis due to sensitive organisms usually in combination with probenecid (Gray's regime). Useful against sensitive coliforms but many are now resistant and *Klebsiella*, *Enterobacter*, *Serratia* and *Pseudomonas* spp. are constitutively resistant. Many strains of *Haemophilus influenzae* and *Moraxella catarrhalis* are also resistant.

Preparations available

Oral and parenteral

Usual adult dose

1–2 g i.v. every 8 h
0.5–1 g p.o. every 8 h

Pharmacology

Well absorbed orally if given before food, and excreted in the bile and urine. Excretion inhibited by probenecid, the combination recommended for the oral maintenance therapy of endocarditis.

Reference

Gray IR. The choice of antibiotic for treating endocarditis. *Quarterly Journal of Medicine* 1975;**44**:449–458

Monitoring

Not required

Side effects

Gastrointestinal intolerance is common: nausea is more common than diarrhoea. The opposite is true for ampicillin which is less well absorbed. Hypersensitivity reactions include rash, either maculopapular or urticarial, fever and bronchospasm. Less commonly, vasculitis, neutropenia, interstitial nephritis, anaphylaxis and angio-oedema and rarely bone marrow suppression causing leucopenia may occur.

Development of a generalised erythematous rash (which may be severe) is common in glandular fever caused by Epstein-Barr virus but this will not recur if the antibiotic is used on a later occasion.

Contraindications

Patients known to have had a type 1 (anaphylactoid) hypersensitivity reaction to any penicillin. A rash associated with glandular fever will theoretically not recur when the patient has recovered and is rechallenged with amoxicillin.

Drug interactions

Synergistic activity with aminoglycosides against both Gram-positive and Gram-negative bacteria. Concomitant use of probenecid delays excretion.

Similar drugs

Ampicillin has no advantage over amoxicillin. It kills bacteria less quickly and is less well absorbed. Esters of ampicillin (talampicillin and pivampicillin) have minor advantages over ampicillin but no advantage over amoxicillin.

See also co-amoxiclav, a combination of amoxicillin and clavulanate, a β-lactamase inhibitor.

References

Pichichero ME and Pichichero DM. Diagnosis of penicillin, amoxycillin and cephalosporin allergy: reliability of examination assessed by skin testing and oral challenge. *Journal of Pediatrics* 1998;**132**:137–143

Canafax DM, Yuan Z, Chonmaitree T, Deka K, Russlie HQ, Giebink GS. Amoxicillin middle ear fluid penetration and pharmakokinetics in children with acute otitis media. *Pediatric Infectious Diseases Journal.* 1998;**17**:149–156

AZITHROMYCIN

An azalide antibiotic acting at the same site as erythromycin which has a broader spectrum of activity (eg including *Haemophilus influenzae*), is active against *Mycobacterium avium-intracellulare* but has strange pharmacokinetics. Treatment is given for a short while: a single dose is effective against many sexually transmitted causes of genital ulcer disease and treatment for three days is probably sufficient for most other infections. There is no evidence that azythromycin is excreted.

Useful references

Journal of Antimicrobial Chemotherapy 1990;**25**(suppA):1–126
Journal of Antimicrobial Chemotherapy 1993; **31**(suppE):1–197
Mazzei T, Surrenti C, Novelli A, Crispo A, Fallani S, Carla V, Surrenti E, Periti P. Pharmacokinetics of azithromycin in patients with impaired hepatic function. *Journal of Antimicrobial Chemotherapy* 1993;**31**:(SuppE)57–63

BENZYL-PENICILLIN — SEE PENICILLIN

CARBENICILLIN

The first useful anti-pseudomonal penicillin has been replaced by ticarcillin: anti-pseudomonal penicillins were superceded by ureido-penicillins (eg azlocillin, now no longer available), acylaminopenicillins (eg piperacillin), anti-pseudomonal cephalosporins and fluoroquinolones. Ticarcillin is used with a β-lactamase inhibitor (clavulanate) as 'Timentin'. (*see Journal of Antimicrobial Chemotherapy* 1989;**24**(supplB):1–226.).

CEFOTAXIME

Antibiotic group

Second generation cephalosporin with a broad spectrum of activity, useful penetration of the CSF but poor against anaerobes and staphylococci.

Spectrum

Excellent activity against coliforms but not most *Pseudomonas* spp. Useful for meningococcal and *Haemophilus influenzae* infections and theoretically active against sensitive Gram-positive infections such as *Streptococcus pneumoniae*. The activity against anaerobes is poor.

Clinical usefulness

Severe Gram-negative infections and meningitis; some penicillin-resistant pneumococcal infections.

Preparations available

Parenteral only. (Intravenous infusion is preferred and intramuscular injection is possible though poorly tolerated).

Usual adult dose

1–2 g 8-hourly

Pharmacology

40% protein bound, well-distributed in tissues and excellent penetration into the CSF. It also crosses the placenta. Most is eliminated as unchanged drug and metabolites (generated in the liver) in the urine; good concentrations are achieved in bile and 20% may be recovered from the faeces.

Monitoring

Not necessary

Side effects

Allergy and effects on bowel flora, including, occasionally, pseudomembranous colitis. Very high blood levels (especially in renal failure) are associated with encephalopathy.

Contraindications

Allergy

Drug interactions

Excretion affected by ureidopenicillins.

Other similar drugs

Cefoxitin (better anti-anaerobe activity than other cephalosporins) and cefotetan (cephamycins), cefoperazone (some activity against *Pseudomonas aeruginosa*); cefotetan and cefoperazone are associated with antabuse-like effect and cause reduced prothrombin (caution with warfarin); ceftriaxone (pharmacokinetics suitable for once-daily dosing and preferred by some paediatricians for the management of meningitis; also useful as a third line drug for the eradication of carriage of *Neisseria* spp.). Cefoxitin is more active against anaerobes than other cephalosporins and is not inactivated by most extended spectrum β-lactamase (cephalosporinases).

   Cefpodoxime proxetil and cefixime are orally active and have a similar spectrum to other second-third generation cephalosporins. Absorption of the former is enhanced by food but decreased by antacids.

References

Journal of Antimicrobial Chemotherapy 1990;**26**(supplA):1–83

Neu H. Third generation cephalosporins: safety profiles after 10 years of clinical use. *Journal of Clinical Pharmacology* 1990;**30**:396–403.

Nau R, Prange HW, Muth P, Mahr P, Menck S, Kolenda H, Sorgel F. Passage of cefotaxime and ceftriaxone into cerebrospinal fluid of patients with uninflamed meninges. *Antimicrobial Agents and Chemotherapy* 1993;**37**:1518–24

Scholz H, Hofmann T, Noack R, Edwards DJ and Stoeckel K. Prospective comparison of ceftriaxone and cefotaxime for the short term treatment of bacterial meningitis in children. *Chemotherapy* 1998;**44**:142–147

Chavanet P, Dalle F, Delisle P, Duong M, Pechinot A, Buisson M, D'Athis P, Portier H. Experimental efficacy of combined ceftriaxone and amoxycillin on penicillin-resistant and broad-spectrum-resistant *Streptococcus* infection. *Journal of Antimicrobial Therapy*. 1998;**41**:237–246

CEFTAZIDIME

Antibiotic group

Third generation (antipseudomonal) cephalosporin.

Spectrum

As for cefotaxime but includes sensitive strains of *Pseudomonas aeruginosa* and arguably less active against Gram-positive organisms.

Clinical usefulness

Severe Gram-negative sepsis, for example in neutropenic patients and those with resistant nosocomial infections. (It is the drug of choice in melioidosis.)

Preparations available

Intravenous only

Usual adult dose

2 g 8-hourly

Pharmacology

Excellent distribution into virtually all tissues and crosses the blood-brain barrier. The dose must be reduced in renal failure.

Monitoring

Not necessary.

Side effects

Allergic reactions and interference with gut flora leading to diarrhoea. Occasional encephalopathy and some photosensitivity.

Contraindications

Allergy

Drug interactions

Incompatible with aminoglycosides in solution.

Other similar drugs

Cefoperazone (a cephamycin with antabuse-like activity and effects on prothrombin) has similar activity but is somewhat less active against *Pseudomonas aeruginosa*. It has no advantages.

Reference

Rains CP, Bryson HM, Peters DH. Ceftazidime: an update of its antibacterial activity, pharmacokinetic properties and therapeutic efficacy. *Drugs* 1995;**49**:577–617

CEFUROXIME

Antibiotic group

Second generation cephalosporin: cefuroxime axetil is bioavailable orally and cefuroxime sodium must be given parenterally either intramuscularly or intravenously.

Spectrum

Active against most Gram-negative aerobic organisms except *Pseudomonas* spp. It is not inactivated by TEM β-lactamases produced by coliforms, *Haemophilus influenzae* and *Neisseria gonorrhoeae* which would inactivate amoxicillin. It is less active than first generation orally-active cephalospor-

ins against Gram-positive organisms. This particularly applies to enterococci and streptococci which are not inhibited *in vivo* and perhaps also to
Staphylococcus aureus.

Clinical usefulness

Useful for definitive treatment of Gram-negative sepsis and for the empirical
therapy of community- and hospital-acquired sepsis and for surgical
prophylaxis. However, widespread use has led to a gradual increase in the
risk that nosocomial pathogens will be resistant. An alternative treatment for
gonorrhoea.

An oral preparation allows parenteral to oral switch of the same agent
established in treatment of Gram-negative infection, where it is thought
necessary to continue during the recovery phase.

Preparations available

Cefuroxime axetil tablets.
Cefuroxime sodium injection.

Usual adult dose

Orally:125–250 mg 6 hourly
Intravenously:1.5–3.0 g 8-hourly

Pharmacology

The oral form is quite well absorbed especially with food reaching peak
serum levels after 3–4 h.

The intravenous form is rapidly and widely distributed in most tissues.
50% is plasma bound. Inadequate levels are achieved in the CSF except
perhaps when the meninges are inflamed. Excreted unchanged in the urine
and there are low concentrations in the bile.

Reference

Mendelman PM, Chaffin DO, Krilov LR, Kalaitzoglu G, Serfass DA,
Onay O, Wiley EA, Overturf GD, Rubin LG. Cefuroxime treatment
failure of non-typable *Haemophilus influenzae* meningitis associated with
alteration of penicillin-binding proteins. *Journal of Infectious Diseases*
1990;**162**:1118–23

Monitoring

Not required

Side effects

As for all cephalosporins: hypersensitivity and gastrointestinal upset including occasional pseudomembranous colitis.

Contraindications

Hypersensitivity.

Drug interactions

None significant. Synergy with aminoglycosides.

Other similar drugs

Cefixime and cefpodoxime proxetil have a similar spectrum and are orally active.

References

Emmerson AM. Cefuroxime axetil. *Journal of Antimicrobial Chemotherapy* 1988;**22**:101–104.
Graber H, Arr M, Magyar T, Ludwig E. Microbiologic and clinical studies with cefuroxime. *International Journal of Clinical Pharmacology Therapeutics and Toxicology* 1983;**21**:399–403
Donn KH, James NC, Powell JR. Bioavailability of cefuroxime axetil formulations. *Journal of Pharmacological Science* 1994;**83**:842–844
Vogel F, Droszcz W, Vondra V, Reisenberg K, Marr C, Staley H. Sequential therapy with cefuroxime followed by cefuroxime axetil in acute exacerbations of chronic bronchitis. *Journal of Antimicrobial Chemotherapy* 1997;**40**:863–871

CEPHALEXIN

Antibiotic group

Representative first generation orally-active cephalosporin

Spectrum

Activity against sensitive coliforms and some Gram-positive bacteria (staphylococci) but generally inactive against streptococci, enterococci, many *Klebsiella*, *Enterobacter* and *Serratia* spp. and all *Pseudomonas* spp..

Clinical usefulness

Urinary tract infections with sensitive organisms. Cephalosporins are not effective in serious staphylococcal infections.

Preparations available

Capsules and oral suspension

Usual adult dose

500 mg every 6 or 8 hours

Pharmacology

Well absorbed but absorption delayed by food. 50% plasma bound. Widely distributed but not into the CSF. Most excreted unchanged in the urine and very high concentrations are achieved. Dose reduction in renal failure.

Monitoring

Not necessary

Side effects

As for all cephalosporins: rashes and gastro-intestinal disturbance including occasional pseudomembranous colitis.

Contraindications

Allergy or infections with resistant organisms.

Drug interactions

None stated

Other similar drugs

All oral cephalosporins are more or less similar. They include cefadroxil (absorption less affected by food and and less protein-bound than cephalexin), cephradine, cefaclor (more active than cephalexin against *Haemophilus influenzae* but possibly more likely to cause allergic reactions on repeated administration), cephalothin and cephazolin (parenteral only).

Reference

Wise R. The pharmacokinetics of the oral cephalosporins — a review. *Journal of Antimicrobial Chemotherapy* 1990;**26**(suppl E):13–20

CHLORAMPHENICOL

Antibiotic group

Unique structure originally obtained from a fungus but now produced synthetically.

Spectrum

A broad spectrum of activity including Gram-positive and -negative aerobes and anaerobes.

Clinical usefulness

In many parts of the world remains the drug of choice for typhoid fever and bacterial meningitis. Sometimes prescribed for brain abscess, preferably with metronidazole. Eye drops and ointment commonly used for conjunctivitis. May be indicated in some unusual infections. The drug is bacteriostatic *in vitro* but may appear bactericidal *in vivo*, for example in typhoid fever. Some strains of *Salmonella typhi* are now resistant. Where available, third generation cephalosporins (eg cefotaxime and ceftriaxone) are favoured over chloramphenicol in paediatric meningitis.

Preparations available

Chloramphenicol palmitate: orally active
Chloramphenicol sodium succinate: for intravenous use.

Usual adult dose

500–1000 mg every 6 hours.

Pharmacology

Chloramphenicol base is bitter. Palmitate is hydrolysed in the gut and absorbed as chloramphenicol.

Monitoring

May be required in babies to ensure adequate blood levels and to exclude toxicity.

Side effects

Bone marrow suppression is a consistent dose-related effect but the drug also rarely causes idiosyncratic fatal bone marrow aplasia. Haemolysis occurs with G6PD deficiency. Very high doses cause shock, vomiting and abdominal discomfort particularly in babies ('grey' syndrome).

Contraindications

Liver disease. Babies need monitoring.

Drug interactions

Antiepileptics may increase (phenobarbitone) or decrease (phenytoin) chloramphenicol levels. Cimetidine may enhance the tendency to aplasia. Paracetamol increases the half-life of chloramphenicol and the latter may interfere with oral contraceptives.

Other similar drugs

Thiamphenicol has no advantages over chloramphenicol.

References

Shann F, Barker J, Poore P. Chloramphenicol alone versus chloramphenicol plus penicillin for bacterial meningitis in children *Lancet* 1985;**ii**:681–683
Shann F. Chloramphenicol for meningitis and pneumonia. *Lancet* 1986;**i**:507
Mermin JH, Townes JM, Gerber M, Dolan N, Mintz ED, Tauxe RV. Typhoid fever in the United States, 1985–1994: changing risks of international travel and increasing antimicrobial rsistance. *Archives of Internal Medicine* 1998;**158**:633–638

CIPROFLOXACIN

Antibiotic group

4-fluoroquinolone

Spectrum

Broad but perhaps most useful against Gram-negatives.

Clinical usefulness

Sepsis with sensitive coliforms and pseudomonads. Some activity against mycobacteria such that quinolones may be used as part of a multi-drug regimen in resistant infections. Very useful in the management of enteric (typhoid) fever.

Preparations available

Tablets, suspension and intravenous solution.

Usual adult dose

200 mg po 12 hly, 500 mg iv 12 hly.

Pharmacology

Well absorbed after oral administration. Widely distributed but not very high concentrations obtained in respiratory secretions from conventional doses.

Reference

Vance-Bryan K, Guay DR, Rotschafer JC. Clinical pharmacokinetics of ciprofloxacin. *Clinical Pharmacokinetics* 1990;**19**:434–461

Monitoring

Not necessary; reduce dose in severe renal failure.

Side effects

Nausea, vomiting and diarrhoea. Headache and hyperactivity, insomnia and nightmares. Photosensitivity and hypersensitivity rashes. Rare effects on the kidneys include interstitial nephritis, and on the marrow include thrombocytopenia and clotting interactions. Degenerative disease of the growing ends of long bones occurs in puppies. Acute tendinitis may occur in man exacerbated by steroids.

Contraindication

In children, reserve for serious infections and withold in pregnancy or nursing mothers.

Reference

Schaad UB, Abdus Salam M, Aujard Y, Dagan R, Green SD, Peltola H, Rubio TT, Smith AL, Adam D. Use of fluoroquinolones in pediatrics: consensus report of the International Society of Chemotherapy commission. *Pediatric Infectious Diseases Journal* 1995;**14**:1–9

Drug interactions

Avoid magnesium- or aluminium-containing antacids and iron (reduced absorption). Potentiates the action of theophylline.

Other similar drugs

Nalidixic acid preceded fluorinated quinolones but had a role only in the management of urinary infection. Many other fluoroquinolone derivatives have been manufactured. Ofloxacin is more active *in vitro* but is less well absorbed. Newer quinolones are sought which have better anti-Gram positive activity. Of these, moxifloxacin is soon to be available.

References

Ciprofloxacin: major advances in intravenous and oral quinolone therapy. *American Journal of Medicine* 1989;**87**(suppl 5A):1S–287S
Ciprofloxacin — defining its role today. *Journal of Antimicrobial Therapy* 1990;**26**(suppl F):1–193.
Anonymous. Fluoroquinolones reviewed. *Drug and Therapeutics Bulletin* 1993;**31**:69–72.
Sanchez-Carrillo C, Cotarelo M, Cercenado E, Vicente T, Blazquez R, Bouza E. Comparative *in vitro* activity of sparfloxacin and eight other antimicrobial agents against clinical isolates of non-tuberculous mycobacteria. *Journal of Antimicrobial Chemotherapy* 1996;**37**:151–154

CLINDAMYCIN

Antibiotic group

Lincosamine: protein synthesis inhibitor acting at at a similar site to erythromycin.

Spectrum

Broad-spectrum particularly against many anaerobes and Gram-positive aerobes (staphylococci and streptococci) but not against enterococci *in vivo*. Active against *Mycoplasma hominis*. Active against some protozoa (eg *Toxoplasma gondii* and *Babesia microtii*) and fungi (eg *Pneumocystis carinii*).

Not significantly active against Gram-negative organisms.

Clinical usefulness

Very effective orally absorbed agent for staphylococcal and streptococcal infections and those where there is likely to be a combination of anaerobic and aerobic organisms (eg mouth flora). Deep-seated infections with *Staphylococcus aureus* (especially osteomyelitis). Favoured in the USA as broad spectrum anti-anaerobic and anti-Gram-positive agent (eg as part of the treatment for intra-abdominal sepsis). Useful as topical treatment of acne and bacterial vaginosis. Has been used in the treatment and prophylaxis of toxoplasmosis and *Pneumocystis* pneumonia in AIDS. (It is not well tolerated in AIDS patients.)

Immune function

Appears to enhance phagocytosis and polymorphonulear neutrophil function.

Reference

Skoutelis AT, Lianou PE, Bassaris HP. *In vivo* potentiation of polymorpho-nuclear leukocyte chemotaxis by clindamycin. *Infection* 1993;**21**:321–323

Preparations available

Oral and parenteral.

Topical preparations available for the skin (acne) and vagina ('anaerobic vaginosis').

Usual adult dose

150–600 mg 6-hourly.

Pharmacology

Well absorbed from the gut so there is no pharmacological advantage in giving the drug parenterally. Food may delay absorption but does not affect total clindamycin absorbed. Well distributed in tissues, especially bone and abscesses. Some topical clindamycin may be absorbed.

Monitoring

Not required.

Side effects

Mild gastro-intestinal disturbance, particularly nausea. Hypersensitivity. The first antibiotic to be clearly associated with pseudomembranous colitis. For this reason, whereas it was very generally used in the 1970s for minor staphylococcal sepsis, it is now reserved for serious infections. However, this drug is probably no more likely to cause this side-effect than many others in common usage. Pseudomembranous colitis has been associated with topical clindamycin.

References

Borriello SP and Larson HE. Antibiotic and pseudomembranous colitis. *Journal of Antimicrobial Chemotherapy* 1981;**7**(suppl A):53–62
Anand A, Bashey B, Mir T, Glatt AE. Epidemiology, clinical manifestations and outcome of *Clostridium difficile*-associated diarrhea. *American Journal of Gastroenterology* 1994;**89**:519–523
Kreisel D, Savel TG, Siler AL, Cunningham JD. Surgical antibiotic prophylaxis and *Clostridium difficile* positivity. *Archives of Surgery* 1995;**130**:989–993
Parry MF, Rha C-K. Pseudomembranous colitis caused by topical clindamycin. *Archives of Dermatology* 1986;**122**:583–584

Contraindications

Pre-existing diarrhoea. Previous pseudomembranous colitis. Hypersensitivity.

Drug interactions

Incompatible with many alkaline drugs and those inactivated at low pH: eg aminophylline, ampicillin, ceftriaxone, phenytoin.

Other similar drugs

Lincomycin is only bioavailable parenterally and is obsolete.

References

Review: Clindamycin in the 1980s. *Journal of Antimicrobial Chemotherapy* 1981;**7**(suppl A):1–85
Blais J, Tardif C, Chamberland S. Effect of clindamycin on intracellular replication, protein synthesis and infectivity of *Toxoplasma gondii*. *Antimicrobial Agents and Chemotherapy* 1993;**37**:2571–2577
Queener SF, Bartlett MS, Richardson JD, Durkin MM, Jay MA, Smith JW. Activity of clindamycin with primaquine against *Pneumocystis carinii in vitro* and *in vivo*. *Antimicrobial Agents and Chemotherapy* 1988:**32**: 807–813

CO-AMOXICLAV

Antibiotic group

β-lactam (amoxicillin) plus β-lactamase inhibitor (clavulanate) combination.

Spectrum

Broad spectrum including many anaerobes. The clavulanate increases the spectrum to include many organisms which would otherwise be resistant to amoxicillin by the production of β-lactamase (eg. penicillin-resistant *Staphylococcus aureus*).

Clinical usefulness

Useful for empirical therapy of urinary and upper and lower respiratory tract infections. Some coliforms and strains of *H. influenzae* are resistant by mechanisms other than β-lactamase production (eg target change or permeability) and co-amoxiclav will offer no advantage over amoxicillin against these.

Preparations available

A wide range of different sized tablets, a suspension and intravenous solution.

Usual adult dose

375 mg tablet (250 mg amoxicillin plus 125 mg clavulanate) given three or four times per day.

Pharmacology

Good parallel absorption of both components, not significantly affected by food. Rapid renal clearance.

Monitoring

Not applicable

Side effects

Allergic reactions as for amoxicillin. Gastrointestinal disturbance. Alteration of prothrombin time, cholestatic jaundice (both rare).

References

Committee on Safety of Medicines. Cholestatic jaundice with co-amoxiclav. *Current Problems* 1993;**19**:2
Thompson JA. Risk factors for the development of amoxicillin-clavulanic acid associated jaundice. *Medical Journal of Australia* 1995;**162**:638–640.
Garcia Rodriguez LA, Stricker BH, Zimmerman HJ. Risk of acute liver injury associated with the combination of amoxycillin and clavulanic acid. *Achives of Internal Medicine* 1996;**156**:1327–1332

Contraindications

Allergy

Drug interactions

Caution with anti-coagulants.

Other similar drugs

Other combinations of β-lactam-β-lactamase inhibitor include ticarcillin-clavulanate and piperacillin-tazobactam.

References

Clavulanate/β-lactam antibiotics: further experience. *Journal of Antimicrobial Chemotherapy* 1989;**24**(suppl B):1–226.
Todd PA and Benfield P. Amoxycillin/clavulanic acid: an update of its antibacterial activity, pharmacokinetic properties and therapeutic use. *Drugs* 1990;**39**:264–307.

CO-TRIMOXAZOLE

Antibiotic group

A combination of folic acid synthesis antagonists, sulphamethoxazole and trimethoprim.

Spectrum

Broad spectrum, no useful activity against anaerobes.

Clinical usefulness

Established in the treatment of urinary and respiratory infections. Useful for *S. aureus* infections (eg. osteomyelitis) if the isolate is sensitive. First-line treatment of *Pneumocystis carinii* pneumonia. Occasional use in brucellosis, typhoid and other rare infections. The sulphonamide component is important in the treatment of nocardiasis (but there is no evidence that co-trimoxazole is better than sulphonamide and perhaps the best treatment is sulphonamide plus amikacin).

Preparations available

Oral combination tablets (standard): 80 mg trimethoprim and 400 mg sulphamethoxazole
 Double dose tablets, various dispersible tablets and suspensions, intravenous infusion.

Usual adult dose

For ordinary infections: 2 standard tablets twice daily but for *Pneumocystis carinii* pneumonia, two double-dose tablets twice per day. A single standard dose is a useful test of cure for uncomplicated urinary infections.

Pharmacology

Both components are well and rapidly absorbed irrespective of food.

Monitoring

Sulpha levels can be measured in AIDS patients and should be less than 200 mg/L. (The time of the sampling is not important once steady state has been achieved).

Side effects

Hypersensitivity rashes are quite common, especially in AIDS. Severe Stevens-Johnson syndrome can occur. Although these are usually attributable to the sulpha component, such rashes can also occur with trimethoprim alone.

Contraindications

Known allergy. Porphyria. There is a view that the addition of sulphonamide confers no significant advantage over trimethoprim but the latter alone is not very good for treating pneumococcal infections. Other side effects are standard for all broad spectrum antibiotics: gastrointestinal intolerance, pseudomembranous colitis and candidal overgrowth.

Drug interactions

Enhance warfarin activity by displacement from plasma binding. Similar problem of sulpha displacing bilirubin from albumin theoretically enhancing the risk of kernicterus in the newborn. Potentiation of sulphonylureas.

Other similar drugs

Many synthetic sulphonamides were produced but have now fallen out of favour.

References

Committee on Safety of Medicines. Revised indications for co-trimoxazole (Septrin, Bactrim, various generic preparations). *Current Problems* 1995;**21**:6

Fischl MA, Dickinson GM, LaVoie L. Safety and efficacy of sulfamethoxazole and trimethoprim chemoprophylaxis for *Pneumocystis carinii*. *Journal of the American Medical Association* 1988;**259**:1185–89.

DOXYCYCLINE

Antibiotic group

Preferred form of tetracycline

Spectrum

Broad spectrum of activity including many Gram-positive and -negative bacteria. *Mycoplasma* spp., *Chlamydia* spp., ureaplasmas, *Brucella* spp. Modest anti-mycobacterial activity.

Clinical usefulness

Not useful for treating conventional pyogenic infections as tetracyclines are generally bacteriostatic against sensitive strains. Tetracyclines were classically associated with the development of 'antibiomas' in staphylococcal abscesses. However, remains very valuable for treating intracellular infections with the organisms mentioned above, rickettsial infections and legionellosis. Effective against most causes of atypical pneumonia. Commonly used in genitourinary medicine clinics and gynaecological patients for treating *Chlamydia trachomatis*. Non-specific urethritis, pelvic inflammatory disease and chronic prostatitis may also respond. Acne (minocycline preferred).

Many *Haemophilus influenzae* strains remain sensitive so tetracyclines remain valuable for treating acute exacerbations of chronic obstructive airways disease if antibiotic treatment is thought to be necessary.

Preparations available

Oral in the form of capsules and dispersible tablets.
(Intravenous preparation is available).

Usual adult dose

200 mg p.o. followed by 100 mg p.o. daily

Pharmacology

Well absorbed. Absorption less affected than tetracycline by calcium, iron and food. Most is protein bound in the circulation, widely distributed in tissues. 40% is excreted through the kidneys, the rest through the liver and it can be given safely in renal failure. Long half-life allows once-daily dosage.

Monitoring

Not required.

Side effects

Oesophageal ulceration may occur if tablets are not swallowed properly. Gastrointestinal effects are common including dry mouth and dysphagia. Candidal overgrowth is common but hypersensitivity is less common than with β-lactams. Excretion affected by liver impairment. Some photosensitivity. Tetracyclines are chelated in bone and are deposited in developing teeth causing discoloration. They should therefore be avoided in pregnancy and in children up to the age of 6y. Rare side-effects include raised intracranial pressure and myopia, haemolytic anaemia and other haematological disturbances.

Contraindications

Porphyria. Pregnancy and childhood.

Drug interactions

Tetracyclines are incompatible with many other drugs in solution. They may be chelated in the stomach if given with antacids or iron. Tetracyclines enhance warfarin activity and may reduce efficacy of the contraceptive pill.

Other similar drugs

Minocycline: preferred in acne
Demeclocycline: used for inappropriate ADH secretion.

Tetracycline, oxytetracycline and chlortetracycline: much cheaper than doxycycline but the latter has very substantial advantages making the earlier preparations obsolescent.

References

Saivin S and Houin G. Clinical pharmacokinetics of doxycycline and minocycline. *Clinical Pharmacokinetics* 1988;**15**:355–366.
Eady EA, Jones CE, Gardner KJ, Taylor JP, Cove JH, Cunliffe WJ. Tetracycline-resistant propionibacteria from acne patients are cross-resistant to doxycycline, but sensitive to minocycline. *British Journal of Dermatology* 1993;**128**:556–560
Eady EA, Cove JH, Holland KT, Cunliffe WJ. Superior antibacterial action and reduced incidence of bacterial resistance in minocycline compared to tetracycline-treated acne patients. *British Journal of Dermatology* 1990;**122**:233–244

ERYTHROMYCIN

Antibiotic group

Macrolide, protein synthesis inhibitor.

Spectrum

Gram-positive aerobic bacteria and many causes of atypical pneumonia and genito-urinary infections (eg *Chlamydia* spp., *Mycoplasma* spp. (though not *M. hominis*), *Legionella* spp.). In general, less active against Gram-negative organisms except for parvobacteria such as *Brucella* spp., *Neisseria* spp. and *Haemophilus* spp.. Not useful clinically against anaerobic bacteria. Modest anti-mycobacterial activity.

Clinical usefulness

Valuable alternative to penicillins for treating staphylococcal and streptococcal infections. Typical and atypical pneumonia. Pelvic inflammatory disease. Legionellosis and other unusual infections including rickettsioses.

Preparations available

Erythromycin base is inactivated by acid. Various salts, esters and microparticles in enteric coating are available.

Erythromycin lactobionate or gluceptate are available for intravenous injection.

Usual adult dose

Oral: 250 mg 6 hly or 500 mg 12 hly
Intravenous: 1 g 6 hly

Pharmacology

Food may delay the absorption of some preparations but not others. Most is excreted in the bile. Erythromycin does not get into the CSF but otherwise it is widely distributed in tissues. In the blood a high proportion is protein bound. It crosses the placenta and gets into breast milk.

Monitoring

Not required

Side effects

Causes minor gastrointestinal side effects in a high proportion of patients. Mostly this is simply nausea but some patients may get hepatitis. The intravenous solution causes local phlebitis. Erythromycin enhances gut motility. Rapid infusion of erythromycin may cause cardiac dysrhythmias.

Contraindications

Hypersensitivity or severe intolerance.

Drug interactions

Erythromycin interferes with the metabolism of many drugs by its interference with cytochrome P450. Important among these are warfarin, corticosteroids, some antiepileptics (eg phenytoin and carbamazepine).

Other similar drugs

Clarithromycin and azithromycin (an azalide) have a similar spectrum of activity but enhanced activity against some Gram-negatives (eg *Haemophilus* spp.) and *Mycobacterium avium intracellulare*. In general they also have better pharmacokinetic and toxicity profiles. Many derivatives of erythromycin have been developed.

References

Eady EA, Ross JI, Cove JH. Multiple mechanisms of erythromycin resistance. *Journal of Antimicrobial Chemotherapy* 1990;**26**:461–465.

Periti P, Mazzei T, Mini E, Novelli A. Adverse effects of macrolide antibacterials. *Drug Safety* 1993;**9**:346–364.

Perez-Trallero E, Urbieta M, Montes M, Ayestaran I, Marimon JM. Emergence of *Streptococcus pyogenes* strains resistant to erythromycin in Gipuzkoa, Spain. *European Journal of Clinical Microbiology and Infectious Diseases*. 1998;**17**:25–31;

FLUCLOXACILLIN

Antibiotic group

β-lactamase-resistant beta-lactam.

Spectrum

Active against penicillin-sensitive organisms but solely used against penicillin-resistant staphylococci or against penicillin-sensitive organisms (eg *Streptococcus pyogenes*) when associated with a β-lactamase producer such as *Pseudomonas aeruginosa*.

Clinical usefulness

Only used for treating significant staphylococcal infections. Its usefulness is now limited by the widespread development of methicillin- (and therefore flucloxacillin-) resistant *Staphylococcus aureus* (MRSA).

Preparations available

Intravenous and oral

Usual adult dose

Intravenous: 0.5–2 g 6 hly
Oral: 250–500 mg 6 hly

Pharmacology

It is well absorbed orally and diffuses well into many body fluids and tissues. It does not penetrate well into pus and bones so should be given together with another active agent with better penetration properties such as fusidic acid. Flucloxacillin will prevent the emergence of resistance to the latter.

Monitoring

Not required

Side effects

Hypersensitivity reactions as for penicillin. Gastrointestinal intolerance, particularly oesophagitis is common when high doses (>500 mg 6 hly) are taken orally. Hepatitis and cholestatic jaundice may occur with increased frequency in prolonged use (more than 2 weeks) and in elderly patients. Interstitial nephritis is a rare side-effect.

Reference

Fairley CK, McNeil JJ, Desmond P, Smallwood R, Young H, Forbes A, Purcell P, Boyd I. Risk factors for development of flucloxacillin associated jaundice. *British Medical Journal* 1993;**306**:233–235 (and **307**:1179)
Committee on safety of medicines. Flucloxacillin jaundice. *Current Problems* 1992;**35**

Contraindications

Patients known to have type 1 hypersensitivity reaction to any penicillin. It should be used with caution in porphyria.

Drug interactions

Synergistic activity with aminoglycosides against staphylococcal infections.

Drug resistance

The *mec*A gene (in *S. aureus* and coagulase negative staphylococci) codes for a novel penicillin binding protein which does not bind to methicillin and its congeners. Resistance may also occur by other mechanisms.

Other similar drugs

Cloxacillin and nafcillin are less well absorbed than flucloxacillin when given orally.

FUSIDIC ACID

Antibiotic group

Fusidane: a unique structure

Spectrum

A broad-spectrum antibiotic effective against many Gram-positive organisms including staphylococci, corynebacteria and *Bacillus* spp. and many anaerobes. Also active against *Mycobacterium tuberculosis* though not used in anti-tuberculosis regimens.

Clinical usefulness

Fusidic acid has particular value in the treatment of deep-seated or complex *S. aureus* infections. In combination with other anti-staphylococcal agents such as flucloxacillin, it is useful in the treatment of staphylococcal osteomyelitis and endocarditis. Its usefulness is limited by the purported emergence of resistance if used on its own.

Fusidic acid inhibits the replication of several viruses *in vitro* but has not been found to be clinically useful.

Preparations available

Oral tablet and suspension and intravenous infusion. Topical preparation available for cutaneous infection

Usual adult dose

Oral and intravenous: 500 mg 8 hly.

Pharmacology

It is well absorbed from the gastrointestinal tract and penetrates well into tissues particularly bone. It is metabolised in the liver. Minimal post-antibiotic effect.

Monitoring

Liver function tests should be monitored regularly while on treatment.

Side effects

Mild gastrointestinal upsets such as gastritis if taken orally, rashes and reversible jaundice. Intravenous infusion may cause thrombophlebitis and more likely to cause jaundice than the oral preparation. Granulocytopenia is a rare side-effect. The topical preparation may cause local hypersensitivity (contact dermatitis).

Immunological effects

Thought to be mildly immunosuppressive and tried in uveitis, Behçet syndrome and multiple sclerosis.

Contraindications

Use with caution in severe liver impairment.

Drug interactions

No major drug interactions, but use with caution in combination with other antibiotics such as rifampicin which have similar biliary excretion pathway, as accumulation of either drug may occur. Gradual induction of cytochrome P450 system over 28 days.

Other similar drugs

None available

References

Taburet AM, Guibert J, Kitzis MD, Sorensen H, Acar JF, Singlas E. Pharmacokinetics of sodium fusidate after single and repeated infusions and oral administration of a new formulation. *Journal of Antimicrobial Chemotherapy* 1990;**25**:23–31

Eykyn SJ. Staphylococcal bacteraemia and endocarditis and fusidic acid. *Journal of Antimicrobial Therapy* 1990;**25**(SupplB):33–38

Jensen T, Lanng S, Faber M, Rosdahl VT, Hoiby N, Koch C. *Journal of Antimicrobial Therapy* 1990;**25**(supplB):45–52

Hoffner SE, Olsson-Liljequist B, Rydgard KJ, Svenson SB, Kallenius G. Susceptibility of mycobacteria to fusidic acid. *European Journal of Clinical Microbiology and Infectious Diseases* 1990;**9**:294–297

Bendtzen K, Diamant M, Faber V. Fusidic acid, an immunosuppressive drug with similar functions to cyclosporin A. *Cytokine* 1990;**2**:423–429

Gentamicin

Antibiotic group

Aminoglycosidic aminocyclitol

Spectrum

Active against some Gram-positive and most Gram-negative aerobic bacteria. It has poor activity given alone against streptococci including enterococci and pneumococci, and no activity against anaerobes.

Clinical usefulness

Widely used for the treatment of serious Gram-negative infections. It has synergistic activity with β-lactam antibiotics (penicillins and cephalosporins) and this is used in the treatment of endocarditis and other Gram-positive infections and severe Gram-negative sepsis. Prophylaxis for urinary tract manipulations.

Preparations available

Intravenous or intramuscular

Usual adult dose

Loading dose — 2 mg/kg followed by 1.0–1.5 mg/kg daily in 3 divided doses.
Alternatively: 5–7 mg/kg intravenously as a single dose given once daily.
    The dosage interval is modified in renal failure by monitoring serum levels.

Pharmacology

Not absorbed from the gastrointestinal tract. Widely distributed in tissues particularly in the kidneys but distribution into the CSF and bronchial secretions is poor. It is excreted almost entirely as active form in the urine with a small amount in the bile.

Monitoring

When using a multiple daily dose, gentamicin is monitored by taking peak and trough serum levels around the third or the fifth dose, to detect accumulation which could result in toxicity of the drug. Trough levels (taken prior to the next dose) should be less than 2 mg/L and peak levels (taken one hour after the dose) should be between 4–8 mg/L. Currently with once daily dosing a single blood sample should be taken at any time between 6–14 h after the infusion and the predicted dose interval derived from the Hartford nomogram.

References

Erdman SM, Rodvold KA, Pryka RD. An updated comparison of drug dosing methods. Part III: aminoglycoside antibiotics. *Clinical Pharmacokinetics* 1991;**20**:374–388

Begg EJ, Barclay ML, Duffull SB. A suggested approach to once-daily aminoglycoside dosing. *British Journal of Clinical Pharmacology* 1995;**39**:605–609

Barza M, Ionnidis JP, Cappelleri JC, Lau J. Single or multiple daily doses of aminoglycosides: a meta-analysis. *British Medical Journal* 1996;**312**: 338–345

Lacy MK, Nicolau DP, Nightingale CH, Quintiliani R. The pharmacodynamics of aminoglycosides. *Clinical Infectious Diseases* 1998;**27**:23–27.

Side effects

Ototoxicity, vestibular and auditory damage and nephrotoxicity are dose-dependent side-effects of all aminoglycosides. The risk is increased in renal failure and by co-administration of other potentially toxic drugs like vancomycin. Rarely hypomagnesaemia occurs on prolonged used. Pseudo-membranous colitis is a rare effect. Attribution of side effects is sometimes difficult because aminoglycosides are rarely given alone.

Contraindications

Aminoglycosides should be used with caution in renal impairment, infants and the elderly. They are contraindicated in pregnancy and myasthenia gravis.

Drug interactions

The risk of nephrotoxicity is increased by concurrent use of antibacterials such as vancomycin, antifungals such as amphotericin, cyclosporin and cytotoxics such as cisplatin. Gentamicin enhances the effect of neuromuscular block by botulinum toxin. Aminoglycosides enhance the effect of muscle relaxants and antagonise the effect of cholinergics such as neostigmine and pyridostigmine. Concurrent use of loop diuretics increases the risk of ototoxicity and renal failure.

Other similar drugs

Streptomycin and kanamycin may be used for resistant mycobacterial infections. Netilmicin and tobramycin are popular alternatives to gentamicin. Though arguably less toxic from animal experiments, netilmicin and gentamicin have similar toxicity rates in clinical practice. Tobramycin is more active against *Pseudomonas aeruginosa*.

See Amikacin (largely used for resistant Gram-negative infections and *Mycobacterium avium intracellulare*).

References

Shawar RM, MacLeod DL, Garber RL, Burns JL, Stapp JR, Clausen CR, Tanaka SK. Activities of tobramycin and six other antibiotics against *Pseudomonas aeruginosa* isolates from patients with cystic fibrosis. *Antimicrobial Agents and Chemotherapy* 1999;**43**:2877–2880

Tulkens PM. Pharmacokinetic and toxicological evaluation of a once-daily regimen versus conventional schedules of netilmicin and amikacin. *Journal of Antimicrobial Therapy* 1991;**27**(supplC):49–61

Tange RA, Dreschler WA, Prins JM, Buller HR, Kuijper EJ, Speelman P. Ototoxicity and nephrotoxicity of gentamicin vs netilmicin in patients with serious infections. A randomised clinical trial. *Clinical Otolaryngology* 1995;**20**:118–123

Bernstein JM, Gorse GJ, Linzmayer MI, Pegram PS, Levin RD, Brummett RE, Markowitz N, Saravolatz LD, Lorber RR. Relative efficacy of netilmicin and tobramycin in oncology patients. *Archives of Internal Medicine* 1986;**146**:2329–2934

Begg EJ, Barclay ML. Aminogycosides- 50 years on. *British Journal of Clinical Pharmacology* 1995;**39**:597–603

The Aminoglycoside Resistance Study Groups. The most frequently occurring aminoglycoside resistance mechanisms. Combined results of surveys in eight regions of the world. *Journal of Chemotherapy* 1995;**7**(suppl2):17–30

IMIPENEM

Antibiotic group

Carbapenem (thienamycin), a bicyclic β-lactam compound together with a purpose-designed enzyme inhibitor (cilastatin) which suppresses degradation in the kidney.

Spectrum

Unparalleled breadth of activity against most Gram-positive and Gram-negative, aerobic and anaerobic bacteria (except *Stenotrophomonas maltophilia* which is inherently resistant to carbapenems) and not active against enterococci *in vivo*.

Clinical usefulness

Valuable as empirical antibiotic monotherapy in febrile neutropenic patients with malignancy or haematological diseases (see also ceftazidime, piptazobactam and ciprofloxacin in this role). Because it tends to be active against multi-resistant strains of Gram-negative bacteria, it should probably be reserved for resistant infections. It should not be used for infections with *Enterococcus* spp.

Preparations available

Intravenous only

Usual adult dose

1–2 g (maximum 4 g) daily in 3–4 divided doses.

Pharmacology

Not absorbed after oral administration. Widely distributed in the body and has been found in the saliva, sputum, pleural fluid, synovial fluid and bone. It is partially inactivated by a dehydropeptidase, an orphan enzyme, in the proximal renal tubule into a metabolite which is inactive. Cilastatin is a specific inhibitor of dehydropeptidase.

Monitoring

Not required.

Side effects

Nausea, vomiting, diarrhoea, taste disturbances. The following side-effects are rare: blood disorders, positive Coombs test, rashes, urticaria and fever. Convulsions, confusion and mental disturbances, red coloration of the urine, erythema, pain and thrombophlebitis may also occur.

Contraindications

Allergy and in breast feeding. It should be used with caution in patients who are known to have had hypersensitivity reaction to penicillins, cephalosporins and other beta-lactam antibiotics, those with renal impairment, epileptics and in pregnancy.

Drug interactions

Combined used of carbapenems with aminoglycosides such as gentamicin show synergy against most bacteria including β-lactam sensitive enterococci.

Other similar drugs

Meropenem is not activated in the proximal renal tubule, so does not require the addition of cilastatin. It has an identical safety profile.

References

Buckley M, Brogden RN, Barradell LB, Goa KL. Imipenem/cilastatin: a reappraisal of its antibacterial activity, pharmacokinetic properties and therapeutic efficacy. *Drugs* 1992;**44**:408–444.

Wiseman LR, Wagstaff AJ, Brogden RN, Bryson HM. Meropenem: a review of its antibacterial activity, pharmacokinetic properties and clinical efficacy. *Drugs* 1995;**50**:73–101.

Meropenem: focus on clinical performance. *Journal of Antimicrobial Chemotherpy* 1995;**36**(suppl A):1–223

Behre G, Link H, Maschmeyer G, Meyer P, Paaz U, Wilhelm M, Hiddeman W. Meropenem monotherapy versus combination therapy with ceftazidime and amikacin for empirical treatment of febrile neutropenic patients. *Annals of Haematology* 1998;**76**:73–80

ISONIAZID

Antibiotic group

Unique agent: isonicotinic acid hydrazide. Specific anti-mycobacterial activity

Spectrum

Highly active against *Mycobacterium tuberculosis* and to a variable extent against 'atypical' species such as *M. avium-intracellulare, M. kansasii* and *M. xenopi*. It is never active against *M. ulcerans*.

Clinical usefulness

Together with rifampicin, the most important anti-tuberculosis combination available. It may also be used alone for chemoprophylaxis of contacts of open cases of tuberculosis with sensitive organisms.

Preparations available

Oral (tablets and solution) and intravenous.

Usual adult dose

Usually given orally. For daily regimens: 300 mg po daily and for intermittent regimens: 15 mg/kg po 3 times/week. The dose may be increased in tuberculous meningitis to 600 mg/day in adults.

Pharmacology

Well absorbed from the gastrointestinal tract and widely distributed in body fluids and tissues including caseous tissues. Penetrates well into the CSF and macrophages, having some activity against intracellular tubercle bacilli. It also crosses the placenta. It is metabolised mainly in the liver and is excreted in the urine and also in breast milk.

Monitoring

Not required. Urine can be checked by a simple dipstick test (BBL TAXO INH Test Strips, Becton Dickinson Co, Sparks, MD 21152, USA) as a check on compliance.

Side effects

Isoniazid is rarely given alone, but when it is used for chemoprophylaxis, severe life-threatening reactions are confined to the elderly. In common with rifampicin and pyrazinamide, isoniazid can cause hepatitis. Transient elevation of transaminases is very common in the first month or two of treatment but spontaneous resolution despite continuing treatment implies that some liver disease is actually caused by tuberculosis. Nausea is common but severe nausea and vomiting almost always indicates hepatitis and all the treatment should be stopped. Peripheral neuritis may occur with high doses. Optic neuritis, convulsions and psychotic episodes may occur. These effects on the central nervous system are exacerbated by pyridoxine deficiency so low dose replacement should be given (eg 10 mg daily). Theoretically, high doses of pyridoxine may interfere with antibacterial activity of isoniazid. Hypersensitivity reactions include fever, erythema multiforme, purpurae and agranulocytosis. Rarely, systemic lupus erythematosus like syndrome with arthritis, pellagra, hyperglycaemia and gynaecomastia may occur. Exacerbation of acne is common.

Contraindications

It should be used with caution in hepatic and renal impairment, epilepsy, alcoholism, porphyria, pregnancy and breast feeding.

Drug interactions

It enhance the effect of antiepileptics such as carbamazepine and phenytoin and also diazepam. It increases plasma theophylline concentrations. Antacids reduce the absorption of the drug.

Drug resistance

Deletions or mutations in the *katG* gene which code for catalase-peroxidase in *M. tuberculosis* lead to resistance. Alternatively, the organism can over-synthesize mycolic acids (over-expression of *inhA* gene). Spontaneous mutants are easily selected by using isoniazid alone.

Other similar drugs

No successful derivatives have been developed.

References

Ormerod LP. Chemotherapy and management of tuberculosis in the United Kingdom: recommendations of the Joint Tuberculosis Committee of the British Thoracic Society. *Thorax* 1990;**45**:403–408
Joint Tuberculosis Committee of the British Thoracic Society. Chemotherapy and management of tuberculosis in the United Kingdom: recommendations 1998. *Thorax* 1998;**53**:536–548
Holdiness MR. Clinical Pharmacokinetics of the antituberculosis drugs. *Clinical Pharmakokinetics* 1984;**9**:511–544

LINEZOLID

Antibiotic group

Synthetic oxazolidinone, structurally unrelated to other antibiotic groups, binds to 50S ribosomal unit to prevent formation of the 70S initiation complex.

Spectrum

Gram-positive aerobes; (some activity against Gram-negative anaerobes and mycobacteria).

Clinical usefulness

New drug, bacteriostatic. Active against many resistant bacteria including methicillin-resistant *Staphylococcus aureus* (MRSA) and glycopeptide-resistant enterococci (GRE) and penicillin-resistant pneumococci (PRP). No cross resistance with macrolides. Clinical usefulness not yet defined.

Preparations available

Oral and intravenous (unlicensed)

Usual adult dose

250–375 mg 8 hly or 625 mg 12 hly

Pharmacology

Serum levels approximately 4 mg/L after single dose of 500 mg. Post-antibiotic effect is 2 h. Preliminary studies suggest that twice-daily dosing shuld be satisfactory. So far, oral administration has been limited to continuation phase after initial intavenous initiation.

Monitoring

Not applicable

Side effects

Nausea and diarrhoea (~7%), vomiting (~2%), headache, dry mouth and discoloured tongue, thrush, dyspepsia and transient changes to hepatic enzymes. Minor symptoms: ~9%, drug discontinuation in early clinical trials: ~9%.

Contraindications

None established.

Drug interactions

None established

Other similar drugs

None available

Reference

Dresser LD, Rybak MJ. The pharmacologic and bacteriologic properties properties of oxazolidinones, a new class of synthetic antimicrobials. *Pharmacotherapy* 1998;**18**:456–462

METRONIDAZOLE

Antibiotic group

Nitroimidazole

Spectrum

Antimicrobial activity restricted to organisms which have either entirely or a substantial component of anaerobic metabolism. It has a wide spectrum of activity against both Gram-positive and Gram-negative anaerobic bacteria except for some nonsporulating Gram-positive bacilli and some *Capnocytophaga* species. It also has some activity against a number of protozoa but none against aerobic bacteria.

Clinical usefulness

It is useful in the treatment of infections due to anaerobic bacteria and protozoa, including *Entamoeba histolytica*, *Giardia intestinalis* and *Trichomonas vaginalis* vaginitis. It is also used in the treatment of *Clostridium difficile*-associated pseudomembranous colitis. Topical preparations used in acne and periodontitis.

Preparations available

Oral in the form of tablet and suspension, suppositories and intravenous infusion. Topical preparation for dermatological and dental use.

Usual adult dose

400 mg po 8 hly
1 g pr 12 hly
500 mg iv 8 hly
Large single doses may be given orally

Pharmacology

Well absorbed orally and rectally and is widely distributed in the body including the CSF. It is mainly excreted by the liver.

Monitoring

Not required.

Side effects

Nausea, vomiting and unpleasant metallic taste in the mouth are common. Less commonly, rashes, urticaria, angio-oedema and, rarely, drowsiness, headache, dizziness, depression and darkening of urine may occur. With prolonged use, painful peripheral neuropathy and, on high doses, transient seizures may occur. Carcinogenic in large doses in rats and positive in the Ames mutagenicity tests in *Salmonella*.

Contraindications

It should be used with caution in hepatic impairment, hepatic encephalopathy, pregnancy and breast feeding.

Drug interactions

Concomitant use with alcohol may result in a disulfiram (antabuse)-like reaction. It enhances the activity of anticoagulants such as warfarin and also increases plasma phenytoin levels by inhibiting its metabolism. It may enhance the toxicity of lithium. Phenobarbitone accelerates the metabolism of metronidazole thus reducing the plasma level of the drug whereas cimetidine has the opposite effect.

Other similar drugs

Tinidazole (longer acting, and seemingly preferred for intestinal amoebiasis). Many other imidazole derivatives have been tried.

References

Lamp KC, Freeman CD, Klutman NE, Lacy MK. Pharmacokinetics and pharmacodynamics of the nitroimidazole antimicrobials. *Clinical Pharmacokineticcs* 1999;**36**:353–373

Bergan T, Solhaug JH, Soreide O, Leinebo O. Comparative pharmacokinetics of metronidazole and tinidazole and their tissue penetration. *Scandinavian Journal of Gastroenterology* 1985;**20**:945–950

Bassily S, Farid Z, el-Masry NA, Mikhail EM. Treatment of intestinal *E. histolytica* and *Giardia lamblia* with metronidazole, tinidazole and ornidazole: a comparative study. *Journal of Tropical Medicine and Hygiene* 1987;**90**:9–12

Boonyapist S, Chinapak O, Plenvanit U. Amoebic liver abscess in Thailand, clinical analysis of 418 cases. *Journal of the Medical Association of Thailand.* 1993;**76**:2 43–246

McDonald HM, O'Loughlin JA, Vigneswaran R, Jolley PT, Harvey JA, Bof A, McDonald PJ. Impact of metronidazole therapy on preterm birth in women with bacterial vaginosis flora (*Gardnerella vaginalis*): a randomised, placebo-controlled trial. *British Journal of Obstetrics and Gynaecology* 1997;**104**:1391–1397

MUPIROCIN

Antibiotic group

Unique agent, pseudomonic acid

Spectrum

Gram-positive infections, (a few Gram-negative organisms).

Clinical usefulness

Topical treatment of staphylococcal and streptococcal infections. Eradication of staphylococcal nasal carriage. Active in superficial 'candidosis' though not active as an antifungal agent *in vitro*.

Preparations available

Topical ointment.

Usual adult dose

Apply topically 3–5 times per day

Pharmacology

If given parenterally, it is inactivated rapidly.

Monitoring

Not required

Side effects

Sometimes local intranasal discomfort.

Contraindications

Resistant isolates (currently 30% of epidemic MRSA)

Drug interactions

Nil

Other similar drugs

Nil

References

Janssen DA, Zarins LT, Schaberg DR, Bradley SF, Terpenning MS, Kauffman CA. Detection and characterisation of mupirocin resistance in *Staphylococcus aureus*. *Antimicrobial Agents and Chemotherapy* 1993;**37**:2003–2006.
Cookson BD. Mupirocin resistance in staphylococci. *Journal of Antimicrobial Chemotherapy* 1990;**25**:497–503

NITROFURANTOIN

Antibiotic group

Nitrofurans

Spectrum

Effective against Gram-positive bacteria including enterococci and staphylococci and most aerobic Gram-negative bacteria except *Pseudomonas aeruginosa* and *Proteus* spp.

Clinical usefulness

Only useful for lower urinary tract infections. Frequently used as urinary prophylaxis in children and also in adult females with chronic urinary tract infection.

Preparations available

Oral only.

Usual adult dose

50–100 mg po 6 hly with food.

Pharmacology

It is well absorbed orally and excreted in the urine.

Monitoring

Not required.

Side effects

Nausea, vomiting, anorexia and diarrhoea are common. Acute and chronic pulmonary reactions ('furadantin lung') with fever and eosinophilia, urticaria, rash, pruritis and peripheral neuropathy have been reported. Rarely cholestatic jaundice, hepatitis, pancreatitis, arthralgia, haemolytic anaemia and myelosuppression may occur.

Contraindications

Contraindicated in renal failure, glucose-6-phosphate dehydrogenase deficiency and in porphyria.

Drug interactions

Nitrofurantoin is antagonistic to nalidixic acid *in vitro*. Probenecid reduces the excretion of nitrofurantoin.

Other similar drugs

None available.

References

Holmberg L, Boman G, Bottiger LE, Eriksson B, Spross R, Wessling A. Adverse reactions to nitrofurantoin: analysis of 921 reports. *American Journal of Medicine* 1980;**69**:733–738

Holmberg L, Boman G. Pulmonary reactions to nitrofurantoin. 447 cases reported to the Swedish adverse drug reaction committee 1966–1976. *European Journal of Respiratory Diseases* 1981;**62**:180–189

PENICILLIN

Antibiotic group

Beta-lactam

Spectrum

Active against Gram-positive cocci, in particular streptococci and staphylococci which do not produce penicillinase. It is also active against Gram-negative cocci including meningococci and gonococci. Of the anaerobes, most of the Gram-positive rods (eg clostridia) and cocci (eg peptostreptococci) are sensitive.

Clinical usefulness

Penicillin retains its usefulness for the treatment of serious infections with sensitive bacteria including cellulitis and erysipelas, where the causal organism is predicted to be *Streptococcus pyogenes*. In the UK, it is still the antibiotic of choice in the treatment of meningococcal, invasive gonococcal and pneumococcal infections. Penicillin in combination with gentamicin is important in the managemant of native valve endocarditis, where the causal organism is commonly a streptococcus. It is also used as prophylaxis in patients with a history of rheumatic fever and in splenectomised patients. Long acting preparations are useful in the treatment of syphilis.

Preparations available

Oral: phenoxymethyl penicillin(penicillin V)
IM/IV: benzyl penicillin (penicillin G)
Long acting: eg benzathine penicillin

Usual adult dose

Intravenous: 1.2–2.4 g every 4–6 h
Oral: 250–750 mg 6 hly
Intramuscular injections are very painful.

Pharmacology

Phenoxymethyl penicillin is acid stable but is not particularly well absorbed when given orally. Although it is used for treating sore throats it is inefficient at eradicating *Streptococcus pyogenes*. Intramuscular injections of penicillin preparations are painful, therefore intravenous injections are preferable especially with higher doses. Generally well distributed but does not penetrate into the CSF unless meninges inflamed.

Monitoring

Not necessary

Side effects

Relatively few. Most serious side effects are hypersensitivity reactions, which include maculopapular or urticarial rashes, fever and bronchospasm and, less commonly, vasculitis, neutropenia, interstitial nephritis, anaphylaxis and angio-oedema. Rarely, bone marrow suppression with leucopenia may occur.

Contraindications

Patients known to have had a hypersensitivity reaction to any penicillin.

Drug interactions

Synergistic activity with aminoglycosides against Gram-positive and Gram-negative bacteria. However, they should not be mixed in the same syringe or infusion. Concomitant use of probenecid delays excretion.

Other similar drugs

See also extended spectrum penicillins such as amoxicillin, piperacillin.

References

Pichichero ME, Pichichero DM. Diagnosis of penicillin, amoxicillin and cephalosporin allergy: reliability of examination assessed by skin testing and oral challenge. *Journal of Paediatrics* 1998;**132**:137–143

PIPERACILLIN

Antibiotic group

β-lactam: extended spectrum acylaminopenicillin

Spectrum

An extended spectrum penicillin with activity against *Pseudomonas aeruginosa* and many other Gram-negative bacilli, it also has extended anaerobic activity which encompasses many *Bacteroides fragilis* strains.

Clinical usefulness

Its principle indication is for the treatment of serious infections caused by *Pseudomonas aeruginosa*, but resistance tends to develop within a short period if the drug is used on its own and the organism is not quickly eradicated. Therefore it is recommended that it is used in combination with a β-lactamase inbitor or an aminoglycoside such as gentamicin. Such a combination is very powerful for the management of nosocomial infections in ICU and the haematology unit.

Preparations available

Injection and infusion

Usual adult dose

Intravenous: 100–150 mg/kg daily in divided doses

Pharmacology

It is active only when given parenterally. It does not penetrate the blood-brain barrier well unless the meninges are inflamed. It is well excreted in the bile and urine.

Monitoring

Not required.

Side effects

See penicillin.
Electrolyte imbalance such as hypernatraemia may occur owing to high sodium content, and may be a particular problem in renal or hepatic failure. Thrombophlebitis may result from large doses or prolonged administration.

Contraindications

See penicillin.

Drug interactions

Similar to penicillin: if used in combination with aminoglycosides it has synergistic activity against both Gram-positive and Gram-negative bacteria including *Pseudomonas aeruginosa*.

Other similar drugs

Carbenicillin, the original anti-pseudomonal penicillin
Ticarcillin, derived from carbenicillin and now sold mainly in combination with clavulanate for serious sepsis.
Azlocillin, an anti-pseudomonal penicillin which is not resistant to β-lactamase.
Piperacillin may be combined with a β-lactamase-inhibitor, tazobactam (see below).

References

Fass RJ, Prior RB. Comparative *in vitro* activities of piperacillin-tazobactam and ticarcillin-clavulanate. *Antimicrobial Agents and Chemotherapy.* 1989;**33**:1268–1274.

Mehtar S, Drabu YJ, Blakemore PH. The *in vitro* avctivity of piperacillin/ tazobactam, ciprofloxacin, ceftazidime, and imipenem against multiple resistant Gram-negative bacteria. *Journal of Antimicrobial Chemotherapy.* 1990;**25**:915–919

PIPERACILLIN/TAZOBACTAM

Antibiotic group

β-lactam (extended spectrum ureidopenicillin) and β lactamase inhibitor (tazobactam) in combination.

Spectrum

This combination provides broader activity against β-lactamase-producing Gram-negative bacteria which are resistant to extended spectrum penicillin alone. Enhanced anti-anaerobic activity and active against penicillin-resistant, methicillin-sensitive staphylococci.

Clinical usefulness

It is useful either as a single agent or in combination with aminoglycoside such as gentamicin for empirical antibiotic therapy in febrile neutropenic patients. Valuable for mixed infections including enterococci sensitive to penicillin as these are resistant to cephalosporins and quinolones.

Preparations available

Intravenous

Usual adult dose

Intravenous: 2.25–4.5 g 8 hly

Pharmacology, side effects, contraindications, drug interactions

As for piperacillin. Tazobactam has similar pharmacokinetic behaviour to piperacillin. Neither cross the blood-brain barrier in sufficient quantity to be useful in meningitis.

Monitoring

Not required.

Other similar drugs

'Timentin' (ticarcillin and clavulanate).

References

Piperacillin/tazobactam: a new β-lactam /β-lactamase combination. *Journal of Antimicrobial Chemotherapy* 1993;**31**(suppl A):1–124

Brun-Buisson C, Sollet JP, Schweich H, Briere S, Petit C. Treatment of ventilator-associated pneumonia with piperacillin-tazobactam/amikacin versus ceftazidime/amikacin: a multicenter, randomised controlled trial. *Clinical Infectious Diseases* 1998;**26**:346–354

PYRAZINAMIDE

Antibiotic group

Specific anti-tuberculosis agent. The mechanism of action is not known. The genetic basis of resistance is unknown.

Spectrum

Active against intracellular dividing forms of *Mycobacterium tuberculosis*. *M. bovis* is constitutively resistant. Other species are variably sensitive.

Clinical usefulness

Used in the initial phase of treatment for *Mycobacterium tuberculosis*. It is particularly useful in tuberculous meningitis because of excellent penetration across the blood-brain barrier.

Preparations available

Oral only

Usual adult dose

Daily regimen	under 50 kg — 1.5 g p.o. daily
	50 kg or over — 2 g p.o. daily
Intermittent regimen	under 50 kg — 2 g p.o. 3 times/week
	50 kg and over — 2.5 g p.o. 3 times/week

Pharmacology

Well absorbed from the gastrointestinal tract and metabolised in the liver, it penetrates well into liver, lungs, kidneys, CSF and macrophages, but to a lesser extent into spleen, bone marrow and skeletal muscle. It is excreted in the bile and urine.

Monitoring

Not required.

Side effects

Fever, anorexia, nausea, vomiting, arthralgia, urticaria may occur. A raised uric acid above baseline is a consistent effect and precipitation of gout is not unusual. Liver failure with jaundice and hepatomegaly is an idiosyncratic reaction but may be fatal. Rarely, sideroblastic anaemia occurs.

Contraindications

It should be used with caution in hepatic or renal impairment, diabetes and gout. It is contraindicated in porphyria.

Drug interactions

It has an antagonistic effect with uricosuric drugs such as probenecid.

Other similar drugs

Morphazinamide is an intravenous form valuable for the rare case where the drug cannot be taken orally and its use is considered essential (eg tuberculous meningitis).

References

see isoniazid

QUINUPRISTIN–DALFOPRISTIN

Antibiotic group

Combination of two streptogramin antibiotics, natural products of *Streptomyces* spp. which inhibit protein synthesis. While each separately is bacteriostatic, together they are bactericidal.

Spectrum

Gram-positive organisms including *Staphylococcus aureus* even when resistant to methicillin (MRSA) and some resistant enterococci, especially glycopeptide resistant *Enterococcus faecium*. Strains resistant to quinupristin-dalfopristin in these species is so far rare. Species of *Enterococcus* other than faecium are resistant.

Clinical usefulness

Licensed for the treatment of infections with resistant organisms. Generally used when other agents have failed or are not tolerated.

Preparations available

Intravenous

Usual adult dose

For example 7.5 mg/kg 8 hly

Pharmacology

Elimination half-lives from the blood of quinupristin is about one hour and dalfopristin half an hour. Excretion is through the biliary system into faeces. Diffuses into tissues but does not cross the blood-brain barrier.

Monitoring

Not applicable

Side effects

Arthralgia (~15%), and myalgia, anorexia, nausea and vomiting, local reactions to infusion and rash.

Contraindications

None stated

Drug interactions

Antagonism *in vitro* with ciprofloxacin.

Other similar drugs

Other streptogramins have been under investigation.

Reference

Bayston R, Hamilton-Miller JMT, Hunter PA, Wood MJ, Daly PJ. Quinupristin/dalfopristin-update on the first injectable streptogramin. *Journal of Antimicrobial Chemotherapy* 1997;**39**(suppl A):1–151

RIFAMPICIN

Antibiotic group

Rifamycin acting by binding RNA polymerase and inhibiting transcription.

Spectrum

A very broad spectrum of activity against Gram-positive bacteria including staphylococci and Gram-negative bacteria including meningococci, gonococci, *Haemophilus influenzae*, brucellae and legionellae. It is also active and perhaps most useful for *Mycobacterium* spp.

Clinical usefulness

It is used in combination with other drugs in anti-tuberculosis regimens and the treatment of leprosy. Resistance develops rapidly when rifampicin is used alone. It is also useful to eradicate respiratory carriage of meningococcus and *Haemophilus influenzae*. Valuable for the treatment of *S. aureus* infections in combination, say, with trimethoprim.

Preparations available

Oral in the form of capsule and syrup and intravenous infusion.

Usual adult dose

0.6–1.2 g po or iv daily in 2–4 divided doses (non tuberculous infections) As anti-tuberculosis therapy see Chapter 5 p. 98

Pharmacology

It is well absorbed taken on an empty stomach and widely distributed. Penetration into the CSF is sufficient for activity against tuberculous meningitis, providing other agents such as pyrazinamide are used in combination. Rifampicin is secreted in the respiratory secretions and colours sweat and urine orange-red. It is metabolised mainly by the liver.

Monitoring

Not required.

Side effects

Orange–red discoloration of body fluids such as urine, saliva, tears and soft contact lenses occurs. Gastrointestinal symptoms such as nausea, vomiting, anorexia and diarrhoea, respiratory symptoms such as shortness of breath may occur. Influenza-like symptoms such as chills, fever, dizziness and bone pain may develop in patients who are on intermittent therapy. Other side effects include haemolytic anaemia, thrombocytopenic purpura, eosinophilia, acute renal failure, jaundice, flushing, urticaria, rashes, collapse and shock.

Contraindications

Contraindicated in porphyria and jaundice. It should be used with caution in hepatic dysfunction, pregnancy and breast feeding.

Drug interactions

Promotes the induction of the hepatic enzymes, reducing the effect of conventional doses of several drugs including *oral contraceptives, anticoagulants*, antiepileptics, *corticosteroids*, diazepam, haloperidol, beta-blockers, verapamil, theophylline, thyroxine, cimetidine cyclosporin, triazole antifungals, antidiabetics including sulphonylureas and antibacterials such as chloramphenicol and dapsone.

Resistance

Mutations in the *rpoB* gene may alter the structure of RNA polymerase to prevent binding.

Other similar drugs

Rifabutin active against some mycobacteria resistant to refampicin — can be used as prophylaxis or treatment of *Mycobacterium avium* complex in AIDS. Rifapentin has pharmacokinetic advantages over rifampicin but is not widely used.

References

see isoniazid.

Horgen L, Legrand E, Rastogi N. Postantibiotic effects of rifampicin, amikacin, clarithromycin and ethambutol used alone or in various two-, three- and four-drug combinations against *Mycobacterium avium*. *FEMS Immunology and Medical Microbiology* 1999;**23**:37–44

TEICOPLANIN

Antibiotic group

Glycopeptide

Spectrum

Gram-positive bacteria.

Clinical usefulness

Serious infections due to staphylococci and streptococci. Sometimes also used for trivial infections because patients are allergic to penicillin.

Preparations available

Parenteral: the solution must not be shaken to dissolve. Intravenous administration preferred but the drug may be given intramuscularly.

Usual adult dose

400 mg iv 12 hly (2 doses), then daily (escalated in endocarditis)

Pharmacology

Long half life and excretion through the kidneys.

Monitoring

Not usually necessary. Serum taken one hour after starting the infusion should have a level exceeding 30 mg/L.

Side effects

Hypersensitivity. Rigors occur in ~15% patients. Local thrombophlebitis. Rare side-effects include bone marrow suppression and abnormal liver function.

Contraindications

Previous hypersensitivity.

Drug interactions

Synergistic with aminoglycosides such as gentamicin against Gram-positive infections.

Other similar drugs

Vancomycin.

Reference

Drabu YJ, Blakemore PH. The post-antibioitc effect of teicoplanin: monotherapy and combination studies. *Journal of Antimicrobial Therapy* 1991;**27**(Suppl B):1–7

TRIMETHOPRIM

Antibiotic group

Synthetic folate antagonist: diaminopyrimidine with action on bacterial dihydrofolate reductase.

Spectrum

Broad spectrum of activity against many Gram-positive and Gram-negative bacteria though not *Pseudomonas aeruginosa*.

Clinical usefulness

Useful for treating urinary tract infection in the community. It is becoming less useful for treatment of community acquired chest infections as resistance is found to be high in *Streptococcus pneumoniae*. Its usefulness is possibly increased by combination with sulphonamides.

Preparations available

Oral tablet and suspension. Intravenous slow injection and infusion.

Usual adult dose

Oral: 200 mg 12 hly
Intravenous: 150–250 mg 12 hly

Pharmacology

Well absorbed from the gastrointestinal tract and distributed in most body
fluids. It also penetrates well into the CSF. It is metabolised in the liver but
90% of unchanged form of the drug is excreted in the urine making it a
useful urinary antibiotic. A small amount is eliminated in bile. Not cleared
by any means of renal replacement.

Monitoring

Not required. In renal failure one dose is administered every three days after
appropriate loading.

Side effects

Nausea, vomiting, pruritis, rashes, depression of haemopoiesis and, less
commonly, erythema multiforme and toxic epidermal necrolysis may occur.
It may also cause megaloblastic anaemia.

Contraindications

It should be used with caution in renal impairment, breast feeding and
porphyria and it is contraindicated in severe renal impairment, pregnancy,
neonates and those with blood dyscrasias.

Drug interactions

Trimethoprim enhances the effect of anti-arrhythmics such as procainamide,
anti-coagulants such as warfarin and anti-diabetics such as sulphonylureas.
Hyperkalaemia. It potentiates the antifolate effect of anti-epileptics such as
phenytoin, anti-malarials such as pyrimethamine and cytotoxics such as
methotrexate. There is an increased risk of nephrotoxicity if used
concurrently with cyclosporin.

Other similar drugs

See Co-trimoxazole, a combination of trimethoprim with a sulphonamide,
sulphamethoxazole.

Reference

Nolan T, Lubitz L, Oberklaid F. Single dose trimethoprim for urinary tract infection. *Archives of Diseases of Childhood* 1989;**64**:581–586.

VANCOMYCIN

Antibiotic group

Glycopeptide

Spectrum

Gram-positive bacteria

Clinical usefulness

Mainly for treating staphylococci resistant to methicillin/flucloxacin. An oral preparation is used to treat severe or recurrent pseudomembranous colitis.

Preparations available

Intravenous-slow infusion over one hour or more.

Usual adult dose

1 g 12-hourly or 500 mg iv 6 hly

Pharmacology

Not absorbed from the gastro-intestinal tract. After slow iv infusion, a wide range of half lives is seen (3–11 h). This is increased in renal failure. A simple rule in patients in renal failure who need vancomycin treatment is to repeat a dose when the trough level (measured daily) falls below 10 mg/L.

Monitoring

Trough serum levels (<10 mg/l) and peak taken 2 h after starting infusion.

References

Pryka RD, Rodvold KA, Erdman SM. An updated comparison of drug dosing methods. Part IV: vancomycin. *Clinical Pharmacokinetics* 1991;**20**:463–476

Leader WG, Chandler MH, Castiglia M. Pharmacokinetic optimisation of vancomycin therapy. *Clinical Pharmacokinetics* 1995;**28**:327–342
Sanders NJ. Why monitor peak vancomycin concentrations? *Lancet* 1994;**344**:1748–1750.

Side effects

If infused too quickly, causes generalised histamine release ('red man syndrome'). Local thrombophlebitis. Ototoxicity and renal toxicity are recognised but rarely attributable to vancomycin alone. Renal failure is very common in combinations with aminoglycosides (as in the treatment of endocarditis). Hypersensitivity reactions with fever, rash are very common especially in prolonged therapy but anaphylaxis is rare.

Reference

Sahai J, Healy DP, Shelton MJ, Miller JS, Ruberg SJ, Polk R. Comparison of vancomycin- and teicoplanin-induced histamine release and 'red man syndrome'. *Antimicrobial Agents and Chemotherapy* 1990;**34**:765–769
Polk RE. Anaphylactoid reactions to glycopeptide antibiotics. *Journal of Antimicrobial Chemotherapy* 1991;**27**(suppl B):17–29

Contraindications

Hypersensitivity

Drug interactions

Incompatible with many drugs in solution.

Other similar drugs

Teicoplanin

5

THE CLINICAL USE OF ANTIBIOTICS

Choosing an appropriate antibiotic to treat an infection is rarely difficult and depends on the syndrome, the probable causal organism(s) and the site of infection. However, the choice of antibiotic regime from a large number of possibilities is a personal one, dependent on availability (some may be excluded from a pharmacy formulary), experience and recommendations in the literature. It may be that quite different antibiotics are recommended for the same indication in different hospitals. There is unlikely to be evidence that one is significantly better than another. Differences reflect historical usage and the preference of the microbiologists. Therefore on arrival at a new hospital, take the trouble to find out what is recommended for the common syndromes. The choices of antibiotics for the main disease syndromes given below are merely a guide to current practice. Be prepared to modify empirical therapy as bacteriology information becomes available. Doses given are a guide to use in adults unless specifically stated. Children's doses are given in the paediatric *vade mecum* and local guidelines.

ACUTE FEBRILE ILLNESS PRESUMED BACTERAEMIA

Community acquired sepsis

Consider the cause. The history is most important in determining the source and cause of the infection. Consider pneumonia, urinary tract infection, gall bladder sepsis and meningitis. (Exclude the possibility of malaria and typhoid from travel history). Make sure that all appropriate specimens (blood culture, full blood count, renal and liver function tests) and a chest X-ray have been taken but do not delay giving an antibiotic, and preferably give it intravenously. In the elderly, coliform bacteraemia from the urinary tract or gall bladder is not uncommon. Confusion in the elderly may reflect urinary sepsis, pneumonia or meningitis. Pneumococcal pneumonia is possible at all ages. Meningococcal sepsis will often present clinically before the characteristic purpuric rash develops.

Use your locally recommended choice of broad-spectrum antibiotic:
Possibilities: one of

- a cephalosporin: cefuroxime, cefotaxime, cefriaxone, etc. (reserve ceftazidime for documented *Pseudomonas* sp. and resistant coliforms)
- a penicillin: benzyl penicillin (best for pneumococcal pneumonia), co-amoxyclav, piperacillin
- a fluoroquinolone: ciprofloxacin (200 mg iv 12 hly) or equivalent (not appropriate for pneumonia)
- a carbapenem: imipenem or meropenem (500 mg iv 8 hly); enormous breadth of activity but expensive for use in empirical therapy

ADD
For suspected Gram-negative sepsis:

- an aminoglycoside: gentamicin or equivalent for synergy; (use once daily dosage: 7 mg/kg and assay serum 6–14 h later)

If there is suspicion of bowel involvement, etc.,

- metronidazole (may be given orally, rectally or intravenously). 500 mg po 12 hly

If there is a suspicion of atypical pneumonia:

- erythromycin 500 mg po 12 hly

Hospital acquired sepsis

Consider the source. Check IV lines, chest, any wound, urine, exclude deep vein thrombosis.

This is often intravenous line associated infection, although bacteraemia secondary to urinary tract infections may also occur. Consider changing suspicious lines. Assume Gram-positive infection:

- flucloxacillin 1 g iv 6 hly for 3 to 5 days **or**
- a glycopeptide: teicoplanin 400 mg iv 12 hly for 3 doses followed by 400 mg iv daily; or vancomycin 1 g iv 12 hly (slow infusion, monitor serum levels)
  If Gram-negative infection suspected, add
- an aminoglycoside, eg gentamicin 7 mg/kg iv single dose, serum level 6–14 h later.

Await results of blood cultures and modify treatment.

BONE AND JOINT INFECTIONS

Acute osteomyelitis and septic arthritis

The most common causal organism is *Staphylococcus aureus*. (Consider *Salmonella* spp. in sickle cell disease.) Empirical treatment should be delayed until samples from bone and blood for culture have been collected. Antibiotics may be started in the operating theatre.

Alternatives

- flucloxacillin 1–2 g iv 6 hly **plus** fusidic acid 500 mg po 8 hly, **or**
- clindamycin up to 600 mg iv/po 6 hly, **or**
- erythromycin 1 g iv 6 hly **plus** fusidic acid 500 mg po 8 hly, **or**

For children under five years old, to cover *H. influenzae* and *Staphylococcus aureus*

- amoxicillin 25 mg/kg 4 hly should be added to above regimen, **or**
- co-amoxiclav 250 mg (expressed as amoxicillin) po 8 hly

Await cultures from bone or blood cultures.

Infection of a **prosthetic joint** is usually caused by *S. epidermidis*. If no isolate or the organism resistant to the above antibiotics, give a glycopeptide:

- teicoplanin 400 mg iv 12 hly for 3 doses then 400 mg iv/im daily, **or**
- vancomycin 1 g slow iv 12 hly, change dose according to levels.

An infected prosthesis will usually require removal or revision.

Chronic osteomyelitis

Surgical removal of dead bone (sequestrum) is required. To establish the causative organism, deep biopsy samples should be taken for culture before starting antibiotics. Anti-staphylococcal antibodies may help in the diagnosis.

- flucloxacillin and fusidic acid dosages as above, **or**

Other suitable antibiotics according to sensitivity tests

- cotrimoxazole
- rifampicin and trimethoprim
- clindamycin

Gram-negative infections such as *Salmonella* spp. in sickle cell patients

- ciprofloxacin (consider carefully before using in children)

Choice of antibiotics to be considered as continuation of oral regimens for many months

- flucloxacillin and fusidic acid
- clindamycin
- erythromycin and fusidic acid
- rifampicin and trimethoprim

Monitor response with serial CRP and anti-staphylococcal antibodies (if appropriate).

CARDIOVASCULAR INFECTIONS

Endocarditis

Always consult a microbiologist if endocarditis is suspected. Take three separate blood cultures separated by days (if the patient is not ill) or by hours (if patient ill). Inform lab that endocarditis suspected. Surrogate markers of infection include normochromic, normocytic anaemia, splenomegaly, haematuria, high ESR and CRP and low albumin. Some patients have impaired renal function.

Native valve endocarditis

Assume α-haemolytic *Streptococcus* sp. Empirical treatment:

- benzyl penicillin 1.2 g iv 4 hly **plus**
- gentamicin 80 mg iv 12 hly.

The length of total treatment course is controversial. According to bacteriology results, antibiotic treatment regimen should be continued orally after initial two weeks of parenteral therapy.

If penicillin sensitive streptococcus is isolated:

- amoxicillin 0.5–1.0 g 6 hly **plus**
- probenecid 500 mg 6 hly

Unless fully sensitive, treatment should be continued parenterally for enterococcal endocarditis:

- benzyl penicillin or amoxicillin iv for 4 weeks **plus**
- gentamicin iv for the first two weeks.

Staphylococcus aureus endocarditis usually presents after a short severe illness and the patient may have peripheral purpurae.

- flucloxacillin 2 g iv 6 hly for 4–6 weeks, **plus**
- gentamicin 80 mg iv 8 hly for the first two weeks.

If a good response, substitute fusidic acid 500 mg po 8 hly for gentamicin. If the endocarditis is caused by coagulase negative staphylococcus resistant to methicillin or MRSA:

- teicoplanin 800 mg iv 12 hly for 3 doses then 800 mg daily for 6 weeks, **plus**
- gentamicin 80 mg iv 8 hly for 2 weeks (if isolate is sensitive).

If no organism is isolated, penicillin iv or teicoplanin iv is given for 6 weeks and gentamicin for the first 2 weeks. However, if a good response to penicillin and gentamicin occurs then the oral phase of amoxicillin and probenecid can be tried.

It is difficult to treat endocarditis because the organisms are present in high numbers in a non-replicating phase and are inaccessible to antibiotics. They may also be resistant to commonly used antibiotics. Surgery is indicated for valve destruction with heart failure or failed chemotherapy (organism inaccessible or resistant).

Prosthetic valve endocarditis

Because coagulase negative staphylococcal infection is likely, initial treatment should include

- Teicoplanin 800 mg iv 12 hly for 3 doses, then 800 mg daily, **plus** gentamicin 80 mg iv 8 hly. Treatment is then modified according to microbiological result, **or**
- Vancomycin 1 g iv 12 hly may be used in place of teicoplanin, but renal function should be closely monitored as gentamicin is used concurrently.

Vascular graft infection

Treat as for prosthetic valve endocarditis; surgery is essential for cure.

- Teicoplanin **or** vancomycin plus gentamicin in dosages as above.

CENTRAL NERVOUS SYSTEM INFECTIONS

Acute bacterial meningitis

The definitive diagnosis of meningitis is made by examining CSF in the laboratory. If lumbar puncture is delayed, do a blood culture, routine blood tests, save EDTA blood for PCR for neisserial DNA, and then give an antibiotic. DO NOT DELAY TREATMENT.

Community-acquired meningitis

The choice of antibiotic depends on the age of the patient, on any underlying disease such as otitis, the presence of a ventricular shunt and post-traumatic CSF leak. Intrathecal antibiotics are not needed (except when treating intraventricular shunt infections with vancomycin or gentamicin).

A dose of antibiotic eg. benzyl penicillin 1.2 g in adults (not known to be hypersentive to beta-lactam antibiotics), should be given as soon as possible either intravenously or intramuscularly in a patient with suspected meningococcal meningitis.

In **neonates** use:

- benzyl penicillin 50 mg/kg iv daily in 2 divided doses plus gentamicin 3 mg/kg q12 h.

If *Listeria* suspected, consider:

- amoxicillin 50–100 mg/kg iv daily in divided doses plus gentamicin (dose as above)

If Gram-negative suspected:

- cefotaxime or ceftazidime 25–60 mg/kg iv daily in 2 divided doses

In **infants**:

- benzyl penicillin 75–100 mg/kg iv daily in 3 to 4 divided doses in clinically suspected meningococcal infection **or**

If cause uncertain:

- cefotaxime 100–150 mg/kg daily in 2–4 divided doses, **or**
- ceftriaxone 1 g daily

In **Adults** use:

- benzyl penicillin 1.2 g iv 4 hly **or**
- cefotaxime 2 g iv 8 hly

If allergic to beta-lactam antibiotics:

- chloramphenicol 500 mg iv 6 hly

Note: Antibiotic treatment should be modified according to the culture results of the CSF.

Brain abscess

Surgical drainage is the mainstay of treatment. Antibiotics which may be used:

- chloramphenicol 500 mg po/iv 6 hly plus metronidazole 400 mg po 8 hly, **or**
- benzyl penicillin 1.2 g iv 4–6 hly plus flucloxacillin 1 g iv 6 hly **plus** metronidazole 400 mg po 8 hly

Post-trauma or post-operative cerebral infection

If intracerebral access is available via shunt or reservoir, take ventricular (and possibly lumbar) CSF for bacteriological diagnosis. Consider:

- ceftazidime 2 g iv 8 hly plus vancomycin 10 mg intraventricularly daily.

Ventricular shunt associated infections

Removal of the shunt is necessary for total eradication of infection. Consider results of bacteriology. Regimens recommended include:

- intraventricular vancomycin 10 mg/day
- ceftazidime 2 g iv 8 hly, possibly **with**
- rifampicin 600 mg po/iv 12 hly or trimethoprim 200–400 mg po 12 hly (only as part of a combination regimen)

Antibiotic prophylaxis for head injury

There is no consensus as to the value of any antibiotic prophylaxis, nor which drug is preferable after head injury.

GASTROINTESTINAL INFECTIONS

Food poisoning

Salmonella, Shigella food poisoning
Antibiotic treatment is not usually required and may prolong the carriage. To prevent systemic complications:

- ciprofloxacin 250 mg po 12 hly

Campylobacter food poisoning
Antibiotic treatment is not usually required. If symptoms are severe (bloody diarrhoea and abdominal pain):

- erythromycin 500 mg po 12 hly, **or**
- ciprofloxacin 250 mg po 12 hly

Bacterial dysentery

Antibiotic therapy is indicated for dysentery caused by *Shigella dysenteriae*.

- ciprofloxacin 500 mg po 12 hly **or**
- according to susceptibility of the organism

Enteric fever (typhoid fever)

- ciprofloxacin 200 mg iv 12 hly or 500 mg po 12 hly, **or**
- chloramphenicol 1 g iv 6 hly or 500 mg po 6 hly.

Pseudomembranous colitis (PMC)

Diarrhoea is very common after antibiotic use. It is best treated by stopping the antibiotics.

PMC is a rare life-threatening condition which may be precipitated by virtually any antibiotic. Stools usually contain the toxins for *Clostridium difficile* but a positive test does not prove the diagnosis. The definitive diagnosis is made only by sigmoidoscopy and biopsy.

- Stop all antibiotics

If severe:

- metronidazole 400 mg po 8 hly, **or**
- vancomycin 125 mg po 6 hly.

Continue for at least two weeks in documented PMC, otherwise stop when the diarrhoea stops.

Helicobacter pylori infection

Treatment recommended for patients with duodenal or gastric ulcer at first diagnosis or on relapse. Regimens commonly used are combinations of:

- omeprazole 40 mg po daily or other proton pump inhibitor **plus**
- clarithromycin 250 mg po 8 hly **plus**
- either amoxicillin 500 mg po 8 hly or metronidazole 400 mg po 8 hly
- colloidal bismuth subcitrate (CBS) 120 mg po 6 hly

taken for 7 days. There are other regimens available, therefore advisable to refer to local policy.

GENITO-URINARY AND SEXUALLY TRANSMITTED DISEASES

It is important to confirm the diagnosis, contact trace, treat and follow up patients with suspected sexually transmitted disease, so they should all be referred to a Department of Genito-Urinary Medicine.

Uncomplicated genital gonorrhoea

- amoxycillin 3 g po plus probenecid 1 g po as single dose, **or**

Genital gonorrhoea and if patient is known to have β-lactam allergy or known resistant organism:

- ciprofloxacin 250–500 mg po single dose, **or**
- ceftriaxone 250 mg im, **or**
- spectinomycin 2 g im single dose

All patients with genital gonorrhoea should also receive one of the following to eradicate concomitant *Chlamydia trachomatis* infection:

- doxycycline 100 mg po 12 hly for 7 days, **or**
- erythromycin 500 mg po 12 hly for 14 days **or**
- azithromycin 1 g po single dose.

Complicated cases of gonorrhoea

Seek expert advice. For sepsis and arthritis, prolonged courses of intravenous penicillin are required.

Non-gonococcal urethritis including *Chlamydia trachomatis* infection

- doxycycline 100 mg po 12 hly for 7 days, **or**
- erythromycin 500 mg po 12 hly for 14 days, **or**
- azithromycin 1 g po single dose **or**
- ofloxacin 400 mg po for 7 days

Pelvic inflammatory disease (PID)

- doxycycline 100 mg po 12 hly for 14 days **plus**
- metronidazole 400 mg po 8 hly for 7 days.

Treatment may need to be modified according to microbiological results.

Candidosis

- clotrimazole single 500 mg pessary nocte and 1% cream to vulva, or
- clotrimazole 200 mg pessary nocte for 3 nights and 1% cream, or
- econazole pessary 150 mg single dose and 1% cream.

Investigate cases resistant to treatment to exclude drug resistance or alternative cause of symptoms. Exclude diabetes mellitus, treat partner, withold broad spectrum antibiotics. Try

- fluconazole 150 mg po single dose.

Trichomonas vaginalis

- metronidazole 2 g po single dose, or 400 mg po 12 hly for 5 days, **or**
- tinidazole 2 g po single dose.

'Anaerobic' vaginosis

Diagnosis by positive amine test, presence of clue cells on direct microscopy. Culture microbiology is unhelpful.

- metronidazole 2 g po single dose, **or** 400 mg po 12 hly for 5 days.

UPPER RESPIRATORY TRACT INFECTIONS

Acute otitis media

This is mainly a disease of infants. Symptoms are usually precipitated by virus infections and controlled trials suggest that antibiotics are no better than placebo. Symptomatic treatment is indicated. Acute tympanitis may be due to *Mycoplasma pneumoniae*.

- amoxicillin 500 mg po 8 hly, **or** if allergic to β-lactams
- erythromycin 500 mg po 12 hly.

If no response, take specimens, consider no antibiotics, **or**

- co-amoxiclav 250 mg (expressed as amoxicillin) po 8 hly

Chronic suppurative otitis media (CSOM)

Treatment should be guided by the results of culture of properly taken pus. Useful antibiotics included:

- co-amoxiclav 250 mg (expressed as amoxicillin) po 8 hly, **or**
- clindamycin 150–300 mg po 6 hly, or

- metronidazole 400 mg po 8 hly, **plus**
- either amoxicillin 500 mg po 8 hly or erythromycin 500 mg po 12 hly.

Invasive otitis externa

This is due to *Pseudomonas aeruginosa* and must be treated with systemic antibiotics. Specimens are taken to establish sensitivity of the isolate. Topical treatment may select for resistance.

- ceftazidime 2 g iv 8 hly, **or**
- ciprofloxacin 400 mg 8 hly iv, possibly **with**
- gentamicin, once daily regimen

Oral ciprofloxacin can be used as a continuation regimen once control of the disease has been secured but should not be used as primary treatment for fear of selecting resistance.

Sinusitis

Surgical drainage of pus is important and the choice of antibiotics is as for CSOM, determined by culture results. Chronic sinusitis often involving the ethmoids is frequently associated with anaerobic colonisation and responds well to regimens including

- metronidazole 400 mg po 8 hly, **or**
- clindamycin 150–300 mg po 6 hly.

Pharyngo-tonsillitis

Exclude glandular fever by checking the full blood count (FBC) and monospot. Culture for Group A *Streptococcus pyogenes*.

- penicillin V 500 mg po 6 hly, **or**
- amoxicillin 500 mg po 8 hly, **or**
- erythromycin 500 mg po 12 hly.

Note the increasing risk of resistance in Group A streptococci to erythromycin. An initial im injection of benzyl penicillin hastens recovery. Long courses of oral penicillin are needed to eradicate the organism, which may be inaccessible to antibiotics.

Pertussis

Antibiotics do not hasten recovery from the symptomatic illness of pertussis. For eradication of the organism from the nasopharynx:

- erythromycin 500 mg po 12 hly.

LOWER RESPIRATORY TRACT INFECTIONS

Acute bronchitis

Most infections are viral, but if secondary bacterial infection is suspected:

- amoxicillin 500 mg po 8 hly, **or**, if allergic to β-lactams:
- erythromycin 500 mg po 12 hly, **or**
- doxycycline 200 mg po daily.

Modify treatment according to culture results (e.g. if resistant *Haemophilus influenzae* or *Staphylococcus aureus* isolated).

Pneumonia: community-acquired

The most common causes of community acquired pneumonia are *Streptococcus pneumoniae* followed by atypical pneumonia caused by *Mycoplasma pneumoniae*. DO NOT DELAY TREATMENT.

- benzyl penicillin 1.2 g iv 4–6 hly, **or**
- cefuroxime 1.5 g iv stat followed by 750 mg iv 8 hly, **plus**
- erythromycin 500 mg po 12 hly

Penicillin-resistant strains of *S. pneumoniae* respond to high dose iv penicillin.

Pneumonitis/bronchiolitis in children

This is often due to viruses such as *respiratory syncytial virus* (RSV) in infants (<1 year). In children under 5 years old, *Haemophilus influenzae* type b may be the cause but this is less frequent since the implementation of immunisation. It is conventional to give an antibiotic such as:

- cefuroxime, **or**
- cefotaxime

Legionnaires' disease

Mild illness:

- erythromycin 500 mg po 12 hly

Severe illness:

- erythromycin 1 g iv 6 hly, **plus either**:
- rifampicin 600 mg orally or iv 12 hly **or**
- ciprofloxacin 200 mg iv 8 hly

Cystic fibrosis

Viral infections usually precipitate acute exacerbations. Antibiotic resistance (e.g. in *Burkholderia cepacia*) is an increasing problem. Empirical therapy could be directed towards the last positive culture but antibiotics should be modified according to the sputum culture result. If pseudomonads are present, use either:

● ceftazidime, **or**
● piptazobactam, **or**
● ciprofloxacin (care in children), **plus**
● an aminoglycoside if clinically indicated.

If *Staphylococcus aureus* is isolated:

● flucloxacillin

If MRSA

● teicoplanin **or** vancomycin

Hospital acquired pneumonia

Most often due to coliforms and pseudomonads or *Staphylococcus aureus*, particularly after anaesthesia and in the intensive care unit. Empirical treatment:

● cefuroxime 750 mg iv 8 hly, or
● cefotaxime 1 g iv 12 hly
● co-amoxiclav 1 g (expressed as amoxicillin) iv 8 hly

If pseudomonads or resistant coliforms isolated,

● ceftazidime 2 g iv 8 hly, **or**
● piptazobactam 4.5 g iv 8 hly, **or**
● ciprofloxacin 200–400 mg iv 8–12 hly depending on severity.

For MRSA, add
● a glycopeptide

Aspiration pneumonia

The chosen antibiotics should cover mouth flora including anaerobes and microaerophilic streptococci.

● clindamycin 300–600 mg po or iv 6 hly, **or**
● co-amoxiclav 1 g (expressed as amoxicillin) iv 8 hly, **or**
● metronidazole with amoxicillin or cefuroxime

Tuberculosis

Initial Phase

Drugs		Daily Dose	
	Adult >50 kg	**Adult <50 kg**	**Child**
Rifampicin	600 mg	450 mg	10 mg/kg
Isoniazid	300 mg	300 mg	10 mg/kg
			(Max 300 mg/day)
Pyridoxine*	10 mg	10 mg	10 mg
Pyrazinamide	2 g	1.5 g	35 mg/kg

* or lowest dose available

Continue until drug sensitivities of isolate known, and if fully sensitive, for a minimum of two months.

Continuation Phase

Discontinue pyrazinamide. Continue for a total of six months.

Ethambutol 15 mg/kg per day may be added in the initial phase of treatment if drug resistance is suspected. (eg previous failed treatment).

Drug resistance

A longer course of therapy will be required. The regimen will be tailored to the isolate and the tolerance of the patient. Take expert advice.

Intermittent supervised treatment

This regimen is recommended for patients with poor compliance. Antimicrobials are given three times per week under supervision.

Initial Phase — these drugs are given 3 times per week for a minimum of 2 months.

Drugs	Adult <50kg	Adult >50kg	Child
Rifampicin	600 mg	900 mg	15 mg/kg
Isoniazid	600 mg	900 mg	15 mg/kg
Pyrazinamide	2 g	2.5 g	50 mg/kg

Continuation Phase

If isolate sensitive, stop pyrazinamide. Continue for a minimum total duration of 6 months.

Combination drugs

Rifampicin plus isoniazid combinations are convenient.

Do not use 'Rifater' because the necessary drug ratios cannot be achieved.

SKIN AND SOFT TISSUE INFECTIONS

Inflammation (cellulitis)

If patient hospitalised for cellulitis,

- benzyl penicillin 1.2 g iv 6 hly **plus** flucloxacillin 500 mg iv 6 hly

If allergic to β-lactam antibiotics:

- erythromycin 1 g iv 6 hly or 500 mg po 12 hly, **or**
- a glycopeptide, **either**
  vancomycin 1 g iv 12 hly, **or**
  teicoplanin 400 mg iv 12 hly for two doses and then daily.

Animal and human bites

- benzyl penicillin 1.2 g iv 6 hly, **or**
- amoxicillin 500 mg iv/po 8 hly

Consider adding metronidazole to penicillin or amoxicillin to enhance anti-anaerobe activity. Alternatively, try

- co-amoxiclav 250–500 mg (expressed as amoxicillin) po 8 hly, **or**
- clindamycin 150–300 mg po 6 hly

Actinomycosis

- benzyl penicillin 1.2 g iv 6 hly for 2–6 weeks, followed by
- penicillin V 500 mg po 6 hly for 3–4 months, **or**

If allergic to β-lactams:

- doxycycline 100 mg po daily for 3–4 months.

Necrotising fasciitis

Surgical debridement is essential.

- benzyl penicillin 1.2–2.4 g iv 6 hly **plus**
- metronidazole 500 mg iv 8 hly (or 400 mg po 8 hly or 1 g pr 8 hly), **or**
- clindamycin 300–600 mg po or iv 6 hly.

Gas gangrene

Surgical debridement is essential.

- benzyl penicillin 1.2–2.4 g iv 6 hly, **plus**
- metronidazole 400 mg po or 500 mg iv 8 hly.

Ecthyma gangrenosum

This is a sign of pseudomonal infection (or rarely systemic fungaemia) in neutropenic patients.

- ceftazidime 2 g iv 8 hly, **or**
- ciprofloxacin 200–400 mg iv 8 hly, **or**
- piptazobactam 4.5 g iv 8 hly

plus

- tobramycin 7 mg/kg iv as single daily dose, serum level at 6–14 h after dose.

Modify treatment according to culture results.

URINARY TRACT INFECTIONS (UTI)

Community acquired UTI

Ideally, properly collected midstream urine (MSU) should be cultured before starting antibiotics. If symptomatic:

- trimethoprim 200 mg po 12 hly.

If treatment fails, modify according to culture results.

Hospital acquired UTI

It is not advisable to treat asymptomatic, elderly or catheterised patients for bacteriuria with antibiotics without good reason. For septic patients, take a specimen and start:

- trimethoprim 200 mg po 12 hly, **or**
- cefuroxime 750 mg iv 8 hly, **or**
- ciprofloxacin 250 mg po 12 hly.

Catheterised patients should be given a single dose of antibiotic (e.g. gentamicin 120 mg im or iv) just before catheter change.

6

ANTIMICROBIAL PROPHYLAXIS

Most surgically invasive procedures which involve an encounter with bacteria usually of the normal flora require antibiotic prophylaxis. This is to reduce the risk of sepsis, post-procedural wound infections and other infectious complications. Effective prophylaxis depends on the correct choice of antibiotics, timing and dosage. Antibiotics should be given to patients with infections (eg peritonitis with appendicitis) as *treatment* not prophylaxis and continued appropriately.

TIMING

Effective prophylaxis is achieved only if there is a high concentration of the antibiotic circulating in the interstitial tissues of the operation site at the time of operation. Therefore, parenteral antibiotic prophylaxis should be administered shortly before the start of the operation or procedure. Ideally intravenous antibiotic(s) should be given with induction of anaesthesia. Oral prophylactic antibiotics are usually recommended for operations and procedures which are to be done under local anaesthesia (eg prophylaxis of endocarditis with dental treatment) and this should be given one hour prior to the procedure.

DOSE

Ideally prophylactic antibiotics should be given as a large single dose. At most the antibiotic may be continued for 24 hours if the operation involves drains or insertion of a prosthesis. Continuation of prophylactic antibiotics beyond this time may be detrimental. For prolonged operations a second dose (4–6 hours after the first dose) given intraoperatively has been recommended though there is no evidence of benefit for this practice.

CHOICE OF ANTIBIOTICS

Postoperative and post-procedural infections are usually caused by endo-genous microflora present at the site of the procedure. Therefore the choice of antibiotic should be based on the knowlege of the presence of these organisms at various sites. If a patient does develop a post-operative or post-procedural infection requiring treatment, it is unwise to use the same antibiotics that have been used for prophylaxis, as the organisms are likely to be resistant to these antibiotics due to prior exposure. Many antibiotic regimens have been tried in procedures with a high risk of post-operative sepsis such as large bowel, vaginal or oral surgery. There are no generally agreed protocols but the suggestions given below are acceptable in most units with some modifications.

RISKS

Relatively few patients do develop post-operative sepsis and some do so despite antibiotic use. As a general rule, rates of sepsis are reduced by about 50%. This implies that the majority receive antibiotics unecessarily. The greatest risk of this practice is with unforeseen type I hypersensitivity. However, the anaesthetist should be able to cope with this emergency. More commonly, the patient will have a side effect such as diarrhoea (even pseudomembranous colitis) or rash. Some antibiotics are specifically contraindicated: for example, gentamicin potentiates the effect of suxamethonium and will substantially delay recovery of paralysis. Some patients given an informed choice would rather not have antibiotics for prophylaxis but keep them in reserve in case of sepsis.

SUGGESTED ANTIBIOTIC PROPHYLAXIS PROTOCOLS

Cardiac procedures

Coronary Artery Bypass Grafts (CABG)

First dose to be given at induction of anaesthesia.

- Flucloxacillin 500 mg iv 6 hly for 4 doses **plus**
- Gentamicin 1.5 mg/kg iv followed by 80 mg iv 8 hly for 2 doses.

Valve replacement and other intracardiac surgery

- Flucloxacillin 500 mg iv at induction, then 6 hly for 8 doses **plus**
- Gentamicin 1.5 mg/kg iv at induction, then 8 hly for 6 doses.

A trough gentamicin level should be checked 24 hours after the operation.

Prophylaxis against endocarditis

As recommended by the British Society of Antimicrobial Chemotherapy (May 1992) in patients with either cardiac valve abnormality or previous history of endocarditis who are undergoing dental and urological procedures.

Dental extraction, scaling or periodontal surgery

Under local or no anaesthesia

- Amoxicillin 3 g po 1 hour before procedure under supervision.

If allergic to β-lactam antibiotics or have received a penicillin within the previous month:

- Clindamycin 600 mg po 1 hour before procedure under supervision.

Under general anaesthesia

- Amoxicillin 1 g iv (or im with 2.5 ml of lignocaine 1%) at induction, then 500 mg po at 6 hours, **or**
- Amoxicillin 3 g po 4 hours before anaesthesia, then 3 g po postoperatively, **or**
- Amoxicillin 3 g po plus probenecid 1 g po 4 hours before the procedure.

High risk patients should be referred to hospital

Such patients include those with a prosthetic valve or allergy to or recent administration of penicillin or previous history of endocarditis.

- Amoxicillin 1 g iv plus gentamicin 120 mg iv or im at induction, followed by amoxicillin 500 mg po at 6 hours.

If allergic to β-lactam antibiotics and had received penicillin within the previous month:

- Vancomycin 1 g iv infusion over 100 mins, 1–2 hours before the procedure plus gentamicin 120 mg iv at induction, **or**
- Teicoplanin 400 mg iv plus gentamicin 120 mg iv at induction, **or**
- Clindamycin 300 mg iv over 10 mins at induction, followed by 150 mg po or iv at 6 hours.

Doses for children are adjusted accordingly. For example,

Children <5 years	amoxicillin	quarter adult dose
	clindamycin	quarter adult dose
	gentamicin	2 mg/kg body weight
Children 5–10 years	amoxicillin	half adult dose
	clindamycin	half adult dose
	gentamicin	2 mg/kg body weight
Vancomycin	for children under 10 years	20 mg/kg body weight
Teicoplanin	for children under 14 years	6 mg/kg body weight

Gastrointestinal procedures

Large bowel surgery/appendicectomy

- Cefuroxime 1.5 g iv plus metronidazole 500 mg iv at induction.

If appendix was acutely inflamed, perforated or pus found then treatment is continued as appropriate. The above doses are repeated 8 hly.

Biliary tract procedures

ERCP

The first dose of the prophylactic antibiotic should be given within 30 minutes before the procedure.

- Cefuroxime 750 mg iv 8 hly for 3 doses **or**, if allergic,:
- Ciprofloxacin 200 mg iv or 500 mg po followed by 500 mg po 12 hly for 2 doses.

A single dose probably is sufficient.

Surgery

- Cefuroxime 750 mg iv at induction and 8 hourly for 2 doses, **or**
- Ciprofloxacin 200 mg iv or 500 mg po followed by 500 mg po 12 hly for 2 doses. **or**
- Amoxicillin 500 mg iv with gentamicin 1.5 mg/kg **or**
- Co-amoxiclav 1.2 g iv with induction.

Upper gastrointestinal procedures

- Cefuroxime 1.5 g iv at induction followed by 750 mg iv 8 hly for 2 doses

If anaerobes suspected (local cancer or achlorhydria), add

- Metronidazole 500 mg iv 8 hly for 2 doses may be added to the above regimen.

Gynaecology procedures

Hysterectomy/emergency Cesarean section

- Co-amoxiclav 1.2 g iv at induction.

Orthopaedic procedures

Hip replacement or metal insertion

- Cefuroxime 1.5 g iv at induction, then 750 mg iv 8 hly for 2 doses, **or**
- Flucloxacillin 1 g iv at induction, then 500 mg po 6 hly for 2 doses.

If allergic to β-lactam antibiotics:

- Erythromycin lactobionate 1 g iv (slow infusion) at induction, followed by:
- Erythromycin (Erymax) 500 mg po 12 hly for 2 doses

Amputation for ischaemia

There is a risk of developing gas gangrene from this type of operation. Therefore prophylactic antibiotics are recommended.

- Benzyl penicillin 1.2 g iv at induction and 6 hly for 48 hours.

If allergic to β-lactam antibiotics:

- Metronidazole 500 mg iv at induction, then 8 hly for 2 doses.

Compound fractures

- Tetanus toxoid
- Benzyl penicillin 1.2 g iv at induction, then 6 hly for 2–6 doses.

If allergic to β-lactam antibiotics:

- Erythromycin lactobionate 1 g iv at induction, followed by:
- Erythromycin (Erymax) 500 mg po 12 hly for 2–6 doses, plus, if heavily soiled
- Metronidazole 500 mg iv then 400 mg po 8 hly.

Urology procedures

Minor interventions eg. cystoscopy, urinary catheter change, urodynamics

- Gentamicin 120 mg iv single dose 10 min before procedure.

Endoscopic urology

- Gentamicin 120 mg iv single dose given 10 min before procedure.

Open surgery

If intestinal material is to be used:

- Cefuroxime 750 mg iv plus metronidazole 500 mg iv at induction (or 1 g pr 1 hr before the operation).

Prophylaxis may be continued for a maximum of 3 doses.

Transrectal prostatic biopsy

- Co-amoxiclav 1.2 g iv, **or**
- Gentamicin 120 mg iv plus metronidazole 500 mg iv

Chemoprophylaxis for contacts of certain infections

Exposure to meningococcal meningitis/septicaemia

- Rifampicin 600 mg po 12 hly for 2 days, children 10 mg/kg po 12 hly for 2 days, **or**
- Ciprofloxacin 500 mg po single dose (not recommended for children)

Exposure to Haemophilus influenzae

- Rifampicin 600 mg po daily for 4 days, children 20 mg/kg po daily (maximum 600 mg), **or**
- Ciprofloxacin 250 mg po 12 hly for 3 days (not recommended for children)

Exposure to Corynebacterium diphtheriae (toxigenic strain)

Adults:

- Erythromycin (Erymax) 500 mg po 12 hly for 5 days.

Children up to 2 years:

- Erythromycin 125 mg po 6 hly,

Children 2–8 years:

- Erythromycin 250 mg po 6 hly

Exposure to whooping cough

- Erythromycin 50 mg/kg daily in 4 divided doses for 7 days.

Prophylaxis for splenectomised patients

- Phenoxymethylpenicillin (Penicillin V) 500 mg po 12 hly.

Consider vaccination against pneumococci (and, less importantly, meningococci and *H. influenzae*) before elective splenectomy.

Prophylaxis for rheumatic fever patients

- Phenoxymethylpenicillin (Penicillin V) 250 mg po 12 hly.

7

ANTIBIOTICS IN ALTERED PHYSIOLOGICAL STATES

PRESCRIBING FOR NEONATES

Neonates differ from adults in their response to medication. Accurate dosing is important and should be calculated according to body weight. At this age there is developmental immaturity in most body systems, including inefficient renal filtration, relative enzyme deficiencies and inadequate detoxifying systems, all of which may lead to accumulation of the drug resulting in toxicity. Due to the complexity in dosage calculations for this age group, it is recommended that the reader should refer to the local policy and paediatric *vade mecum.*

PRESCRIBING FOR THE ELDERLY

Many elderly patients are debilitated and have limited renal reserves leading to accumulation of drugs due to slow excretion. They are highly susceptible to nephrotoxic drugs. Elderly patients tend to receive polypharmacy for multiple symptoms. This increases the risk of drug interactions and may potentiate adverse drug reactions. It is therefore necessary to consider carefully whether antimicrobials are absolutely essential before prescribing. For example, if a nephrotoxic antibacterial is to be used, it is appropriate to check whether the patient is already on another nephrotoxic drug that may potentiate the effect, and to check serum creatinine. A good example would be to plan to give gentamicin to a patient on frusemide. Antimicrobials should be reviewed regularly and should be stopped promptly once their purpose is achieved or, as in the case of empirical prescribing, there has been no effect. The absorption of orally administered penicillin may be increased in elderly patients due to relative gastric achlorhydria.

PRESCRIBING FOR PREGNANT AND NURSING MOTHERS (see Table 1)

Almost all antimicrobials cross the placenta in varying concentrations. Similarly they may well be excreted in breast milk of nursing mothers. Therefore it is essential to remember that antibacterial agents in pregnant and nursing mothers may lead to the direct exposure of the drug to the fetus and newborn with attendant toxicity or teratogenicity. For example, the use of nephrotoxic agents such as aminoglycosides and glycopeptides should be used with caution and the levels need to be monitored regularly. Some antibacterial agents are teratogenic in animal studies. These include metronidazole, ethionamide and ticarcillin. Some antibacterials such as the penicillins, cephalosporins and erythromycin are unlikely to be teratogenic and are regarded as relatively safe to be used in pregnancy. The teratogenic potential in others such as rifampicin and trimethoprim are unknown.

Tetracyclines taken in pregnancy cause discolouration of fetal dentition and may also cause acute fatty necrosis of the liver, pancreas and renal damage. The liver damage due to the use of tetracycline may be severe and fatal. Tetracycline in pregnancy and young children stains the secondary dentition as well as the milk teeth.

During pregnancy, the volume of distribution of most drugs is increased implying reduced availability of antibacterials to the tissues. For example, serum levels of a given dose of ampicillin are found to be lower in pregnancy than in a non-pregnant state. This may be due in part to more rapid clearance of the drug and higher doses may need to be considered to achieve a therapeutic blood level. Sulphonamides displace bilirubin from albumin and could theoretically precipitate hyperbilirubinaemia and kernicterus. Aminoglycosides given in pregnancy may cause deafness in the child and other neurological effects. Metronidazole is mutagenic in the Ames salmonella mutagenicity test. Whereas there have been no reports of human birth malformation as a result of its use, it behoves the physician to take enormous care when prescribing for pregnant women and to clearly state the justification in the patient's notes.

Table 1.

The following list of antibacterials may have harmful effects in pregnancy:

Aminoglycosides
- auditory or vestibular nerve damage; greater risk with streptomycin, probably very small with gentamicin and tobramycin
- avoid unless essential in second and third trimester

Azithromycin
- not known to be harmful
- manufacturer advises use only if adequate alternatives not available

Chloramphenicol
- neonatal 'grey syndrome' in third trimester

Ciprofloxacin
- arthropathy in animal studies, avoid throughout pregnancy

Clarithromycin
- not known to be harmful, but manufacturer advises avoid unless absolutely essential

Co-amoxiclav
- no evidence of teratogenicity but manufacturer advises avoid unless essential

Co-trimoxazole
- theoretical teratogenic risk in first trimester, trimethoprim being folate antagonist
- neonatal haemolysis and methaemoglobinaemia in third trimester

Doxycycline – see tetracycline

Ethambutol
- neural tube defects in rodents

Imipenem
- manufacturer advises toxicity in animal studies

Metronidazole
- manufacturer advises avoidance of high dose regimens

Nitrofurantoin
- may produce neonatal haemolysis if used at term

Prothionamide/ethionamide
- mutagenic

Rifampicin
- very high doses are teratogenic in animal studies in the first trimester
- risk of neonatal bleeding may be increased if given in third trimester

Sulphonamide
- theoretically increases bilirubinaemia in neonate

Tetracyclines
- effects on skeletal development in animal studies if given in first trimester
- dental discoloration, maternal hepatotoxicity with large parenteral doses in second and third trimester

Table 1. (continued)

Trimethoprim
- theoretical teratogenic risk in the first trimester

Vancomycin
- little information available
- manufacturer advises avoid unless expected benefit outweighs potential risks

---

PRESCRIBING IN THE PRESENCE OF RENAL FAILURE

Renal excretion is the most important route of elimination of most antibacterials. In the presence of renal impairment, lower doses of antibacterials such as aminoglycosides, glycopeptides, ethambutol and carbapenems, should be used to reduce the development of toxic side effects. Dosage modifications of β-lactam antibiotics including penicillins and cephalosporins, quinolones, folate antagonists and antituberculosis drugs such as isoniazid are needed only in the presence of severe renal failure. Some antibacterials such as nitrofurantoin and tetracyclines (except doxycycline) are contraindicated in renal failure. Recommended dose reductions are indicated in Table 2.

Table 2. Doses of antibacterials for adults recommended in serious infections and in renal failure

Antibiotic	Usual adult daily dose (mg × number of doses per day) (parenteral unless otherwise stated)	Moderate renal failure creatinine clearence 10–50 ml/min¶	severe renal failure creatinine clearence < 10 ml/min
Amoxicillin	500–1000 × 3	500 × 3	250 × 3
*Amikacin	7.5 mg/Kg × 2	single loading dose then monitor; redose when trough < 5 mg/L	
Benzyl penicillin	1200 × 4	75%	50%
Ceftazidime	2000 × 3	1000 daily	500 every 48 h
Cefuroxime	1500 × 3	750 × 2	750 × 2
Cefotaxime	2000 × 3	2000 × 2	Half dose × 3
Ceftriaxone	2000 × 1	no change	no change if liver function satisfactory
Chloramphenicol	500 × 4 po	500 × 4	500 × 4
Ciprofloxacin	400 × 2–3	400 × 2	200 × 2
Clarithromycin	500 × 2	500 × 2	500 × 1

Table 2. (continued)

Clindamicin	300–600 × 4 po	300–600 × 2	300 × 2
*Co-trimoxazole	960 × 2 po	half after 3 days	avoid
Doxycycline	100 × 1 or × 2 po	no change	no change
Erythromicin	500 × 2 po	no change	500 × 1
Ethambutol	15 mg/Kg/day	Avoid	
Flucloxacillin	1000 × 4	no change	no change
Fusidate	500 (po) × 3	no change	no change
*Gentamicin	7 mg/Kg/day, monitor at 6–14 h to	Single dose 3 mg/Kg, then monitor, redose when trough 2 mg/L	Single dose 2 mg/Kg, then monitor
Imipenem	1000 × 3	500 × 3 (>20 ml/min) 500 × 2 (<20 ml/min)	250 × 2
Isoniazid	300 × 1	no change	no change
Meropenem	500 x3	500 × 2	250 × 1
Metronidazole	400 × 3	no change	400 × 2
Nitrofurantoin po	100 × 2 po only	Avoid	avoid
Piperacillin/ tazobactam	4500 × 3	no change	4500 × 2
Pyrazinamide po	1500–2000 × 1	no change	no change
Rifampicin	450–600 × 1	no change	no change
*Teicoplanin every third day	400 × 2 then × 1	Load then 400 alt die	Load then 400
Trimethoprim	200–400 × 2	Reduce to 200 × 1 after 3rd day	100 × 1
*Vancomycin	1000 × 2	Single dose then monitor	Single dose then monitor

Notes

- calculations for creatinine clearance: Lean body mass = 2.3 × every inch over 5 ft added to 50 for males and 45.5 for females. Then the creatinine clearence is (140-age) × lean body mass × 1.23 (male) or 1.04 (female) / serum creatinine (micromol/L)
- For moderate renal failure, complex dose adjustments are recommended for some drugs at different levels of creatinine clearance eg ceftazidime
- If an oral regimen (po) is suggested, this implies that bioavailability is sufficiently good from oral as compared with parenteral administration to treat serious infection. Otherwise no parenteral preparation is available (eg nitrofurantoin)

PRESCRIBING IN THE PRESENCE OF LIVER FAILURE

Although renal excretion is the most frequent route of elimination of majority of the antibacterials, some are metabolised in the liver before excretion. These include macrolides, chloramphenicol, tetracycline, flucloxacillin, fusidic acid, rifampicin, metronidazole and some cephalosporins such as ceftriaxone. Bone marrow suppression due to chloramphenicol is much more likely to occur in patients with impaired hepatic function. Therefore the dosage should be modified in patients with cirrhosis and other severe liver diseases. Some antibacterials such as ampicillin and ciprofloxacin are excreted in high concentrations in the bile. In patients with liver disease or biliary obstruction this effect may be significantly reduced. In liver failure, particular caution should be taken with cotrimoxazole, clindamycin, doxycycline, macrolides, ceftriaxone and fucidic acid.

PRESCRIBING IN THE PRESENCE OF METABOLIC ABNORMALITY

The presence of metabolic disorder such as diabetes mellitus may affect the absorption of antibacterials and drug availability in tissues. Studies have shown that absorption of intramuscularly administered antibacterials may be impaired in diabetics. This is a good reason to use the intravenous route to initiate antibacterial therapy in seriously-ill patients. Certain antibacterials such as chloramphenicol may potentiate the activity of oral hypoglycaemic agents such as sulphonylureas, by inhibiting microsomal activity in the liver. Many antibiotics are contraindicated in porphyrias and a few precipitate haemolysis in G6PD-deficiency. Many antibiotics are contraindicated in porphyrias and a few precipitate haemolysis in G6PD-deficiency (Table 3).

Table 3a. Antibacterial agents considered unsafe in porphyrias

Cephalosporins	Nalidixic acid
Chloramphenicol	Nitrofurantoin
Cycloserine (second-line anti-tuberculosis agent)	Pyrazinamide
	Rifamycins (rifampicin and rifabutin)
Erythromycin	
Ethionamide (second-line anti-tuberculosis agent)	Tetracyclines (including doxycycline)
	Trimethoprim
Flucloxacillin	
Isoniazid	

Table 3b. The following antibacterial agents may precipitate haemolysis in G6PD-deficiency

Definite
Sulphonamides (eg sulphamethoxazole)
Nalidixic acid
Nitrofurantoin

Table 3b. (continued)

Possible
Sulphonamides (eg sulphadimidine)
Ciprofloxacin and norfloxacin
Para-aminosalicylic acid (second-line anti-tuberculosis agent)
Chloramphenicol
(Probenecid)

DRUG INTERACTIONS WITH ANTIBACTERIALS

There are many important drug interactions with antimicrobials which are summarised in Table 4. The most predictable are those with drugs such as rifampicin, tetracyclines, chloramphenicol and macrolides, which enhance or decrease liver metabolism by changes in the cytochrome p450 system. In addition, bacterial synergy or antagonism could be considered a reflection of drug interaction and some examples have been included in the table.

Table 4. Important drug interactions

Drug	Increases effect or levels of	Decreases effect of
β-lactams	Aminoglycosides (synergy)	
Penicillin, amoxicillin		Chloramphenicol (antagonism)
Amikacin	Muscle relaxants	
Aminoglycosides	Muscle relaxants	
Antacids (Al^{++} Ca^{++} Mg^{++} Zn^{++} Fe^{+++} or Bi^{++})	Clarithromycin	Tetracyclines, ciprofloxacin ethambutol, nitrofurantoin (absorption)
Cephalosporins		Coomb's test positive, difficulty with cross match (5%)
Ceftazidime	Renal failure with aminoglycosides	Chloramphenicol
Cefuroxime and cefotaxime	As all cephalosporins	
Chloramphenicol	Warfarin, tolbutamide, phenytoin	
Ciprofloxacin	Alcohol, theophylline, warfarin, cyclosporin	

Table 4. (Continued)

Drug	Increases effect or levels of	Decreases effect of
	(increased creatinine), glibenclamide	
Clarithromycin	Ergot derivatives, cisapride, pimozide, terfenadine (cardiac dysrhythmia), triazolam, midazolam, lovastatin, phenytoin, cyclosporin, theophylline, digoxin, phenytoin, carbamazepine, valproate, omeprazole	Zidovudine Cytochrome p450
Clindamycin	Neuromuscular blocking agents.	
Erythromycin		
Co-trimoxazole	Warfarin, phenytoin, sulphonylureas and digoxin. Thiazides (thrombocytopenia), pyrimethamine (megaloblastic anaemia)	Renal transplantation (decreased renal function)
Doxycycline		Penicillin (antagonism) Barbiturates, phenytoin, carbamazepine, alcohol, oral contraceptives
Erythromycin	see clarithromycin	C p450
Ethambutol		
Flucloxacillin	see penicillin	
Frusemide	Renal and ototoxicity of aminoglycosides	
Fusidate		Gradual induction of C p450 (see rifampicin)
Gentamicin	Muscle relaxants	
Imipenem		
Isoniazid	Phenytoin, warfarin, diazepam	Enflurane, azoles
Metoclopramide	Ciprofloxacin (better absorption)	
Metronidazole	Alcohol (antabuse-like effect), warfarin, lithium,	
Nitrofurantoin		Ciprofloxacin
Opiates		Ciprofloxacin

Table 4. (Continued)

Drug	Increases effect or levels of	Decreases effect of
Paracetamol	Chloramphenicol	
Phenobarbitone		Metronidazole, chloramphenicol
Prednisolone	Isoniazid, ethionamide	
Probenecid	Penicillins, cephalosporins, ciprofloxacin, cilastatin, nitrofurantoin (decreased excretion)	
Piperacillin/tazobactam	Anticoagulants, vecuronium, methotrexate.	
Pyrazinamide	Probenecid	
Rifampicin	Para-aminosalicylic acid, ketoconazole	Warfarin, other azoles, sulphonylureas, oral contraceptives, corticosteroids, phenytoin, diazepam, theophylline, vitamin D, digoxin, methadone, protease inhibitors, cyclosporin
Teicoplanin	Aminoglycosides	
Theophylline		Erythromycin
Trimethoprim	Digoxin, phenytoin, procainamide, other folate suppressants, cyclosporin.	
Vancomycin	Aminoglycosides	

A simple rule: do not mix solutions of any intravenous antibiotics. Penicillin is inactivated with ciprofloxacin or gentamicin, etc.